Where Their Feet Dance

Where Their Feet Dance

English Women's Sexual Fantasies

by Rachel Silver

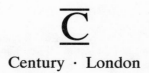
Century · London

Published by Century in 1994

1 3 5 7 9 10 8 6 4 2

Century
20 Vauxhall Bridge Road, London SW1V 2SA

Random House Australia (Pty) Ltd
20 Alfred Street, Milsons Point
Sydney, NSW 2061, Australia

Random House New Zealand Ltd
18 Poland Road, Glenfield
Auckland 10, New Zealand

Random House South Africa (Pty) Ltd
PO Box 337, Bergvlei, South Africa

Random House UK Limited Reg. No. 954009

A CIP catalogue record for this book is available from the British Library

ISBN 0 7126 6000 3

Typeset by SX Composing Ltd, Rayleigh, Essex
Printed and bound in the United Kingdom by
Clays Ltd, St Ives plc

'Dancing in Ireland nightly, gone
To Norway (the ploughboy bridled),
Nightlong under the blackamoor spraddled,
Back beside their spouse by dawn . . .

        . . . who's to know
Where their feet dance while their heads sleep?'

Ted Hughes, 'Witches', *Lupercal*

Contents

Acknowledgements

I would like to thank all the women who contributed their thoughts and fantasies in the preparation of this work.

INTRODUCTION

Introduction

'This is a fantasy that I often think of when I masturbate,' confides my twenty-nine year old neighbour Jessica over a glass of wine, 'and even sometimes when I am making love with my boyfriend. It is a great trigger and even just a brief flash of this fantasy makes me come very quickly. It harks back to my days at an over-zealous religious school.

'I have done something wrong, like not handing in an essay or not turning up for assembly, and am sent to see the headmaster.

'Once inside his study I stand before him as he tells me off, gesticulating wildly and wagging his finger. He begins to talk about God and the devil and bad girls. I yawn, he grabs me by the arm and says that I'm a very disobedient girl. His eyes are flashing with anger. I move closer towards him and kiss him on his large, fleshy mouth. I push him back into the leather chair which stands beside his big desk. And as he sits down hard I climb astride him on his lap and holding his head in both hands whilst also pushing my crotch hard into his lap, I kiss him deep and hard. He pushes me away roughly, saying that I am evil and mad, but against his will I can feel his huge cock getting fatter and fatter until it is very clearly visible through his trousers.

'Standing up now, I tempt and seduce and tease, rubbing my legs and body against him, my little school skirt rising to my waist, and he gets very angry. He flings me to the floor, rips open his trousers, and fucks me very hard with his vast cock, telling me all the while what a dirty temptress and seductress I am, and his eyes blaze as he tells me I am from the devil. His anger turns me on, and I feel so full up with that lovely enormous cock that I feel as if I am in heaven, the best sex I have ever had, and I am degrading him in the process, sucking his strength.

3

'Suddenly he comes, shaking and pushing deeper into me with enormous spasms of come. He is left spent and defiled and with a sticky mess covering his clothes. I am strong and powerful. I stand over him, a seductress, and look down at his gorgeous hulking body with a mixture of disdain and longing.'

Imagery like this, from Jessica's fantasy, is both exciting and at the same time disturbing, and the thought of sharing it with someone else causes her not a little embarrassment.

Twenty years ago, any mention of sex at a casual gathering would have caused an embarrassed silence, but whenever I raised the subject during the writing of this book, the reaction was invariably an animated discussion, on the part of both men and women. In today's liberal moral climate, the emotional confusion aroused by sexual fantasy has emerged from the bedroom and is being debated in public forums everywhere. Quite simply, the subject of women's sexual fantasy is out of the closet.

The fantastical scenario of documenting women's fantasies has been pioneered by Nancy Friday. But there are marked differences in the imagery and descriptions reported by her American subjects, and the English women to whom I spoke in the course of my research. It was wonderfully refreshing to escape from the claustrophobic, straightjacketed *Playboy/Mayfair* language and tone of Friday's work. A great benefit of my approach was that I interviewed people face to face, which allowed the true humour and eccentricity – no doubt on occasion a camouflage for their embarrassment – of British womanhood to emerge, which a pre-prepared questionnaire could never reflect.

My earliest conversations with women to some extent made me reconsider how liberated they really were. Though some had outrageous and lively lustful thoughts, many, if not most of those I spoke to, were initially disappointingly banal. These first research experiences produced certain preconceptions and prejudices, and I began to worry that I might be taking these with me into my interviews. Were many of these women going to tell me they had the classic 'nice girl' rape fantasy, relinquishing responsibility for sexual pleasure? In fact this did not happen, and as I became bolder with my interview subjects so they became bolder with me. And although to some extent my preconceptions about the reticence of the English were confirmed, they were also frequently contradicted, and there were a lot of surprises.

4

The further I went with the interviews the more I learnt to question and draw people out. Initially I often felt protective of their coyness and didn't want to pry, but gradually I discovered that women wanted me to draw out their fantasies and to touch on the notions of meaning and origin. They wanted to reflect on their childhood and adolescence, to be aware of what images excited them most and to discover why this was the case.

I was also concerned that during the interviews they might be telling me only what they considered to be their acceptable fantasies, and not revealing those that they kept in the deepest recesses of their fantasy world. Perhaps predictably, the fantasies told to me by my lesbian contacts – more candid because they'd come out and had confronted their sexuality already – were more provocative and descriptive.

I worried too that the natural reticence of women might be more easily overcome if they were able to describe their fantasies in the anonymity of a letter or a questionnaire. Yet the responses to my advertising and to asking friends to write were curiously less satisfactory than the interviews I was doing, both in the numbers of respondees and in the openness with which they expressed their thoughts. But one such, Marsha, from Newcastle, who described herself as 'forty-three, blonde, voluptuous, attached and a school teacher', was forthcoming and lively in her letter:

'I have so many fantasies, I don't know where to begin. My latest involves my school boys. I invite six of my favourite sixth formers back to my place. I get them drunk (not difficult) and then turn down the lights, and put on a sexy video. I encourage them to undress and when they're really hot and hard (not difficult), I slip into something comfortable – shiny, see-through black lingerie. I lie on the sofa, and get them to stand around me. I flirt, tease and flatter them all in turn, and we start oiling each other's bodies. I pull their penises closer to my face and tell them to pull their pricks over my greedy mouth which parts, pants and kisses. By talking sexily and by licking their pricks I make them start to come – and I smear their virgin spunk all over my body and theirs. Before the last one can come I pull him down on top of me and get him to stuff me, while the rest watch and lick and grope my body.

'By the end of the evening, they've all had their turn and my cunt is full of their spunk, and we all go off to sleep.'

The subject of sex brings out in turn the most retiring and the most outrageous qualities in people. The very notion that women's erotic fantasies exist arouses both vehement disapproval and excited interest. Friends with young children reported that nowadays they were far too tired to fantasise, but they were looking forward to reading the book to give them back some long-lost ideas.

Nancy Friday's books, which are the first to take a serious look at this theme, have helped to place the concept firmly in the open. But as she points out in her most recent book, *Women On Top*, it is an odd time to be writing about sex. 'Not at all like the 1960s and 1970s,' she writes, 'when the air was charged with sexual curiosity, women's lives were changing at the rate of a geometric progression, and the exploration of women's sexuality ranked right up there with economic equality. Today's sexual climate is sombre.'

Although orgies, so much a game of the gilded youth of London's Swinging Sixties, are no longer *de rigueur*, and AIDS casts a very real shadow over indiscriminate lovemaking, the fact is that most women today are free to have the sexual relationship of their choice and to explore the length and breadth of their sexual imagination without shame. Sixties and seventies revolutionaries like Friday herself may well look back and remember dancing naked on the stage of *Hair* and wonder why no one is doing it any more. But the reason is surely not that women have lost interest in sex, but simply that they no longer have to keep proving their right to sexual freedom. Discussing their fantasies openly is part of that new-found freedom.

British women in the 1990s are more sexually and professionally liberated than they have been at any other time in history. We can make choices about being single or being lovers (with male or female partner), wives, mothers or working professionals, extracting what we want out of any combination of these as we like.

Erotica and sexual fantasy are no longer male preserves. Anaïs Nin is no longer a lone voice in the wilderness of women's sexual fantasy. In today's Britain, Madonna's huge best-selling

Sex has effectively exposed all those who wished to remain hidden behind the shop-soiled myth that women must remain modest and ignore their sexual thoughts – assuming that they had any in the first place. Madonna has become the post-feminist contemporary ideal, exemplifying the blatant female sexual identity already loudly proclaimed by leading women's magazines like *Cosmopolitan*, *Marie-Claire*, and the new soft-porn magazines for women.

Sexual fantasy is the subject that women want to talk about now. It is a subject they want to explore to the hilt. As Martin Amis comments in his review of Madonna's book, 'Sex is in the head. And the head has never been so crowded, or so hot, or so noisy.' At London's hottest nightspot, *The Ministry Of Sound*, women are dressing in revealing bras, Janet Reger-style French knickers and thigh-length black leather boots – sexually provocative, but at the same time keeping their distance. They dance in splendid isolation. AIDS and a sexual confidence combine to place the emphasis on alternatives – fantasy, dressing up, telephone sex, masturbation – whether mutual or solitary.

Madonna admits she is turned on by images of homosexual couples of either sex making love. She describes this at length in her book and is photographed participating in her fantasy.

'I love my pussy,' she proclaims. 'It is the summation of my life. My pussy is the temple of learning. Sometimes I sit at the edge of the bed and stare into the mirror . . . Sometimes I stick my finger in my pussy and wiggle it around in the dark wetness and feel what a cock or a tongue must feel when I'm sitting on it . . . ' Madonna, at the age of 34, is one of a generation of women who have grown up unashamed of their bodies. Her fantasies and those of women participating in this book are varied, bold and unashamed. The old, so-called rape fantasies of the pre-liberated nice girl have all but disappeared and been replaced with fantasies involving multiple partners, bondage, S & M, and even such bizarre fantasy scenarios as the image of Madonna nonchalantly hitchhiking naked on a major highway wearing only high heels, a handbag and a cigarette. There is humour as well as eroticism in this upfront sexuality.

Other women are willing to be as candid about their most intimate thoughts, their most delicate susceptibilities, as she is. I

7

talked with women of a variety of ages, from women of twenty to those in their early fifties. As one might have expected, the younger women were generally more open than the older ones, but since all have decided for themselves whether to be in control or to relinquish control, their fantasies are no longer about pretending a lack of responsibility for a guilty secret.

Sarah, a former actress in her late thirties, fantasises about touching herself in public. She imagines herself in exotic locations away from her humdrum daily life. 'I often fantasise that I am on a boat, paddling up a river in China. There are people on the shore, but no one can see that I am masturbating as I move slowly upriver. I don't know if I should admit this, but I actually sit on my bedroom floor wearing a Chinese hat and paddling with a cricket bat. The fantasy seems real to me as I act it out and I come very quickly.'

In my interviews with women, it was not only their sexual imagination that I was interested in, but also the reality of their relationships and real sex life. Thus I hoped to reveal the link between fact and fantasy. Increasingly through the interviews I found I wanted to know whether they wished to live out those fantasies in real life or whether they simply wished to retain them as imagery. What is it that leads us to create such powerful and meaningful fantasy scenarios?

English women have a very different vocabulary and different terms of reference from the Americans of Nancy Friday's work. Class divisions still define people in this country, though clearly not to the extent that they once did. These varying influences do have a marked effect on their sex lives and sexual imagination in terms of language and upbringing.

The last two decades have produced dramatic emotional changes for women. Suddenly, unconstrained feminine eroticism and feminine lust exist without guilt. Women are fantasising alone or whilst having sex with a lover. Defying the notion of sex only being acceptable as part of an emotional relationship, they fantasise about strangers – a man they might never see again.

Nancy Friday concurs, 'After generations of limits, suddenly there were no limits. Sexual freedom was fresh and believable, and women trusted the new images and words of other women saying it was all right to be sexually in control and powerful . . .

and out of this unstructured, limitless erotic ethos, the fantasy of the Great Seductress was born.'

What follows is the result of women being given a chance to give free expression to a central aspect of their lives that has previously remained largely unspoken. English people and English women in particular have always been represented as stereotypically embarrassed by sex and sexual expression. This is of course a myth, the reality being that given the opportunity English women have a rich and surprising fantasy life, all the more interesting and detailed for having been repressed for so long.

THE YOUNGER FANTASIST

The Younger Fantasist

Amanda, Katrina and Caroline are all in their early twenties and attempt to be quite open about their sexuality and sexual fantasies. Amanda, small, dark-haired and voluptuous with a soft, almost childlike voice, is the only one who comes from a family background that was sexually liberal. We talked one morning in a pub where she works as a cleaner, only one of the many jobs she does to earn her way around the world.

Of all the women I interviewed, the younger women were the most spontaneously open in terms of speaking to me about their fantasies. They clearly enjoyed the sex and the associated language, and our encounters seemed quite enjoyable occasions for them. Caroline, a tall, slim and rather self-assured biology graduate was particularly curious to hear what other women had been fantasising about. She explained that she had raised the subject amongst her friends and they had all begun to reveal their sexual fantasies for the first time.

Even Mills and Boon, purveyor of romantic fiction popular amongst younger women, is more frank nowadays, pointed out Amanda, who tends to read these novels as she works. They have launched a new line of sexually explicit stories for the 1990s, to reflect the current interest in women's sexual imagination and fantasy. These new format 'Temptation' romances have all but swept aside the stolen, chaste kiss in favour of sexual realism. Today the fantasy heroines are independent, professional, sexually aware women who travel the world. One such is film agent Molly Hill, who plays sex games with her blindfolded, naked hero and then seduces him while conducting a business negotiation on the telephone. '"Yes . . . I'm . . . I'm a little out of breath from working out." His hand slid beneath her buttocks . . .'

13

All three of these women are quite exhibitionistic, imagining sexual activity in public places where they might well be seen. Caroline fantasises about making love outdoors, 'though not in England, it's too bloody cold.' And the vibrant, forthright Katrina, who works in television production, particularly desires to be pampered and adored, the centre of attention.

Amanda aged 22

I've always wanted to be in bed with four men. They could do anything they wanted to me, though they wouldn't tie me up or anything, and I'd just lie there and enjoy it. I imagine I'm lying there, with one man caressing all the different parts of my body. They can touch me anywhere they want, swapping around. They would be doing everything to me, I wouldn't have to do anything to them, and this would go on for about an hour.

I haven't got a boyfriend at the moment, but I am quite free and relaxed about sex. I'm quite game to try things. I would even want to try out my fantasy if the opportunity came up, though when a friend once asked me to make up a 'three in the bed' with her and her boyfriend I thought, Oh no! I'd have to have been really drunk to say yes. I wouldn't want to remember the next day.

I do like trying out different ideas in my head, though as I haven't got a boyfriend at the moment I try not to do it every day and overcompensate. On reflection, if I was rich and famous and had the time I probably would try out my fantasies.

Another fantasy I often have is about going to bed with Madonna. If I ever was a lesbian then I probably would go to bed with her, because I think she's beautiful – or maybe even if I wasn't. When I was in New York recently I went with friends to quite a few gay clubs, all girls. It's amazing when you go to these places, I didn't know what they were. Here in England most of the women who go to these places are quite butch, but over there they were beautiful, like models. So if I met up with Madonna I probably would sleep with her.

I think that men can get turned on much more quickly than a woman and need the whole element of fantasy much less than women do.

I've always wanted to have a day when I would go and be a stripper. Make a dirty film. It would have to be with somebody that I like, or a film star, not a porn star, but someone like Mel Gibson. He would go down on me and then fuck me. It would be really, really erotic. Being with him would excite me very much, and I like the idea of the film crew being there. I think you just have to switch off from everybody and get into the performance, just get on with it, and then have lots of retakes. I'm quite kinky, actually.

The film *Indecent Proposal* really turns me on. I'd like to sleep with someone like Robert Redford for a million dollars.

I've been to Amsterdam twice, and seen the women standing half-naked and provocative in the red-light district. And I just walk around and wonder what I'd be like standing there. Some of the girls are really stunning, not fat or anything, young girls standing in the windows in a G-string, they don't care.

I don't think I'd tell a boyfriend about my fantasies, it's the sort of thing you might only tell your girlfriends. I know that a lot of men fantasise about having two women, and I'd like to do that and see what the man's face would look like.

I like the idea of the four men fantasy because men usually expect a lot from women, and I just want to lie there and enjoy them caressing me, giving me love. My fantasy isn't dirty, they're not taking turns fucking me or anything. They're touching, stroking and kissing me all over, touching my hair. I'd like them to get really excited, it's exciting for me because it makes me feel so special. If they're good at it, it definitely makes you feel special, the centre of attention. I don't feel guilty about it. I like to choose people, like a few ex-boyfriends and film stars, to be in the fantasy. Nobody that I don't like would be there, only beautiful men with short dark hair, blue eyes, nice firm bodies, nice mouths. They've got to be male, not weeds, nice hairy chests. In the fantasy they are real men. I like to fantasise when I'm on my own, masturbating in bed before I go to sleep at night. It makes you go to sleep with a smile on your face.

I don't get out that much because I work quite hard. I don't really know many men. I just work hard, and I travel and drive a nice car. I'm not that into men at the moment. If I feel like having a bit of sex, obviously I've got to be careful, though casual. I like sex. On the other hand, I really want to settle down and have babies. So there are two different extremes: on the one hand I just want to go out and have fun and travel the world and on the other hand I just want to settle down and have a baby. If I got pregnant now by mistake I'd have the baby. I don't know if that makes me a modern woman or not.

The fantasy where I'm with four men is, I think, my main

one. Often, it takes place in locations other than just in bed, such as on an exotic island, somewhere warm, like the Maldives. We're on the beach and rolling in and out of the sea. Everything happens really naturally and slowly. Lots of loving, and when I tell them the things I want done to me I start to get really excited. I ask them to start from the bottom; they kiss my legs and then kiss the inside of my legs. And one moves up to kiss my neck. And I'm wearing a really sex black lacy body thing, a tiny black G-string tightly underneath. I like to turn them on, the foreplay, seeing them getting excited excites me. I like to watch them getting excited by the things I do. I masturbate in front of them, things like that. With most men it's just kissing and getting on top of each other, and I like to imagine more than that. In my fantasies the men get really excited because I'm so good at the sexy things I do.

I love the idea of sucking cocks and people licking me out. So the men in my fantasy would have to kiss my breasts and lick me out, and we take it in turns and one is sucking my nipples, another sucking my clitoris, then I go down on them in turn, then we do a sixty-nine position where I'm giving them head and they lick me out. A friend of mine actually does things with her boyfriend like being tied up and beaten and masturbating in front of him, which he really loves. I wish I had the guts to carry out some of my fantasies.

Katrina aged 23

I fantasise when I'm with my lover and when I'm on my own. I used to have one fantasy when I was masturbating, it was like a *Carry On* film set in the Restoration, seventeenth century, and I'd be on a great big four-poster bed, and I'd have all these maids around me. I fantasise about women quite a lot. I haven't had a relationship with a member of the opposite sex, but I have had an encounter with a girlfriend. I decided that that's not the way I want to go, but I do fantasise about women. I'm on this bed and there are all these women around me, wearing seventeenth-century maids' costumes, and I'm being pampered. And then there's a queue of men outside, with cocks that are really stiff, and they're completely naked, and they're normally black men, though I've never been to bed with a black man. If I'm not turned on I don't think, I'd like to go to bed with a black man, but if I'm masturbating they come into my thoughts a lot. They're queuing up and they come to the door and I say, yes, no, yes . . . I can have them or turn them away, it's almost like I'm the queen of a castle. In this Restoration scene, in fact, I am the queen of the castle being pampered, deciding which ones I want, and they come in and I say 'turn me on', and they have to do everything, I don't do anything. They have to come on top of me, and they have to turn me on. I'm resisting and they have to pursue it. That was one that I used to have a lot about three years ago.

I used to have another one as well. Most of my fantasies are about being with lots of men. This time I'm in this big champagne glass, a massive big champagne glass, and I've got these athletes climbing up, desperate to get to me.

I'm inside the champagne glass, naked, with lots of cotton wool, and it's all pink, though I hate the colour pink. It's really weird how when you fantasise things are so different from what you really think. I hate the colour pink, and I don't really want to go to bed with a black man, not that I'm racist or anything, but I don't lust after black men except in my fantasies. It's the stereo-typical black man with a big penis I go for, they always have fit bodies and are naturally toned.

So, there are about twenty black men climbing up this massive champagne glass. I'm in the middle and they're on the outskirts of this glass, and they're all crawling over the brim. And the first one that gets his bum into the champagne glass gets to have me, and everybody else drops away. And they're all fighting to get into the champagne glass. It's a proper bowl-shaped champagne glass. And he comes over to me. Most of my fantasies are men doing everything to me – I don't know if that's laziness! But they come and do things to me and I just lie there.

I like softness, so I fantasise about soft things, and small things. I don't really like pain – apart from when I'm really turned on. My boyfriend really likes pain in sex, but I don't. So I think about men kissing me really really softly all over and I like the thought of something really soft and small – I mean my clitoris as well – like when my boyfriend's penis hasn't got completely stiff yet; it tickles me and turns me on when he's soft. And sometimes when I have sex with him I imagine – because my boyfriend is really tall, but he's undeveloped and he hasn't got the biggest penis in the world, he's quite feminine and his chest's really small and undeveloped – so sometimes when we're having sex if he's trying to make me orgasm I fantasise that I'm having sex with a seventeen-year-old public school boy who's a virgin. And that really turns me on, a bloke that's never had sex. I'm teaching him and seducing him. I'm the powerful woman, like when I'm the queen, that's what comes out in my fantasies.

I love the public school boy fantasy. I think it's probably a class thing. I was brought up in a working-class atmosphere and I've always had an attraction to men who've been to public schools – a cut above the rest; perhaps I'd like to be like them. I've never been out with one though, and really I think they're wankers. But in sexual fantasy when I masturbate I like to dominate and overpower a public school boy, which has something to do with the class thing. When I was a kid I always wanted to be one of these rich kids – you see them as rich kids when you're little. That clean-cut look – very short hair, soft skin – really does something for me, especially when I'm having sex. It really cleans things up for me. I used to think that that was really sick, but I don't think about it so much now.

As you get older you hear stories of women going out with younger men, although I'd never go out with younger men. I'd

19

never even consider going out with a seventeen-year-old. I suppose fantasies let you imagine you would do things which you don't accept that you would ever actually do.

The champagne glass fantasy has been my biggest fantasy over the last four years. And also the thought of my body slithering through cotton wool buds. The idea of cotton wool buds touching me all over really turns me on, tickling me. If you imagine a whole lot of cotton wool buds between your legs it's very frustrating because it all gets smaller and there's nothing solid. It's like a small penis or a penis that's not exactly firm – it's so frustrating, because it sort of flops where you don't want it to. I find it so exciting when a guy tries to make you orgasm when he's already come, and he's going soft. It's exciting because it might go really floppy any second; there's that excitement and pressure to get there before there's nothing left there to make you come. It's a wonderful tease, and in a way it reminds me of my public school boy fantasy quite a lot because my boyfriend is so slim and undeveloped – so it comes to mind when we're having sex.

I can look at pictures of the Chippendales and it wouldn't do a thing for me, but if the image came to me in a fantasy it would, the opposite of what I really go for. A real seventeen-year-old public schoolboy wouldn't do a thing for me, but it does during sex. But if I'm on my own masturbating it will always be big strong men, and I have power over them, and they have to do everything I want them to do. I like the idea of black men with bobbly noses rubbing them up against my clit, it really turns me on. I suppose it's because I started masturbating with a teddy bear called Pépé. My mum made me this cuddly toy called Pépé because I wanted another little brother and I couldn't have one. I liked to go to bed with the teddy bear, and that's how I discovered orgasm, from slithering around and cuddling Pépé. Pépé was the same size as me – I was about eleven at the time, and he was a massive big teddy. He used to give me this funny feeling. I'd be rubbing up against him and the funny feeling would come, and that's how I discovered the orgasm. I know a lot of women use pillows the first time they masturbate, but pillows were too set and strong for me, and Pépé was ideal until he was used as Guy Fawkes on the bonfire when I was sixteen. I cried my eyes

20

out, but Mum said it was so ripped and torn. I was brought up in a very strict Catholic family and wasn't told about orgasm or anything. So I thought that when Pépé was burnt I wouldn't get this funny feeling any more. I couldn't believe it when I saw him on the bonfire, it really broke my heart. I felt really wicked about Pépé, a real guilt trip.

When I was at school I was put in the principal group for the school play. I was only thirteen, mixing with sixteen-year-old girls. I was always paranoid that there was a camera in the room. Once it was a girl's birthday and all the girls bought her presents and at one point they took out a big pillow and everyone started laughing. Suddenly they stopped and said 'Oh no, Katrina's in here', because I was the youngest and they felt embarrassed because I shouldn't know about these things. I knew about the pillow, and when they stopped laughing I thought, my God, they all know about my secret of Pépé, and I cried. And nobody understood why I was crying. I was sure that they had all been peeping through my window, and it was a big joke. That's how naive I was at the time. So orgasms were a real guilt trip. My first boyfriend never gave me an orgasm, so I just thought it was something I could do on my own.

At twenty-three I've only actually had sex with two men, and my first experience was nothing to boast about. I've been seeing my present boyfriend for six years now and I suppose we've discovered a lot together. I have told him about my main fantasy, which really is the Restoration fantasy, where I am queen of the castle.

At the castle the women would be seducing me first. I'd have about six women kissing and licking and massaging me, and masturbating with me to turn me on, so that I'm itching by the time the men come. And they have to walk in with such great stiff cocks, they have to be really ready, they're all masturbating outside. It's almost like all of us are at a peak, so when we get together it's like electricity. I play a lot with the idea of them coming inside me and then I push them away and take another one, and they all watch and then it's their turn, it's a real teasing game. I really get off with a real teasing game. And they're actually begging to come back into me, and the more they beg the more I get somebody else, and the more they have to watch. I

21

love the pain of it – the mental torture and the control turns me on so that I can come and come.

Coming from a devout Catholic family meant that I didn't feel in control of my sexuality when I was young, so this whole thing of how I'd be absolutely fantastic, and I am a sex machine and a sex goddess, is a real turn-on for me because it was never like that. I never knew anything. All the girls had sex before I did. I was seventeen when I first had sex. I had this idea that it was that I wanted to be a virgin when I did it with the right person at the right time, but it probably wasn't. It was probably because I was so scared. I remember once lying at school, saying that I'd been fingered when I hadn't, because I felt such a twat. Everyone had done everything and I hadn't done anything.

Now everything is about me being in control. Though I'm quite lazy about sex, I want everything done for me and to me. My boyfriend lives away, and the minute he sees me he wants to get into bed, and I'm not like that at all. He's really highly sexed and I'm not. If he works me into it then I can really let myself go, but if he wants to do something unusual like use chocolate or food I have to be quite worked up; otherwise I'll be thinking, Oh God, it's going to dirty the duvet, and I'll have to clean it tomorrow! Unless I'm pissed or in a really ecstatic mood I won't do it, because it's too messy and sticky. I'd rather just get my head down and go to sleep. I sound quite boring like that, but I suppose my fantasies are more erotic, more sickly, more dirty, a lot more juices rolling around. I love the scene in *Nine And A Half Weeks* where the girl had to eat food she could not see. But if it was me I'd be the one making the man crawl across the floor blindfolded, I'd be the one in control.

I think young women now want to be in control and have the sex they want to have. My mum was brought up to hate sex. She described it to me as the most awful thing ever, and said you should only do it if you want to have children. She hates it. I can imagine her having sex. She'd probably just lie there and let him do it, she'd grit her teeth, she'd hate it that much. Maybe it's also got something to do with the fact that I don't think she ever really loved my dad. I don't think she'd ever admit to herself that she might want to be the leader. She wouldn't enjoy it. It's never been part of her life, she just did it for children. Every time I try and talk to her about sex she says, don't talk about it, it's disgusting. I suppose there's a built-in part of me that sees sex as a weakness, and I see men that really want to have sex as really weak. It makes me want to taunt them, not humiliate them, but make them want me, and be weaker than me. I don't like to be vulnerable. I used not to like to have sex with the light on – showing vulnerability is quite a big thing for me.

I always imagine sex as this wonderful, erotic, juice-swopping experience, but when you actually have it it can just become embarrassing and even comic when you bang into each other or one of you falls off the end of the bed. In fantasy the bed is vast and goes on for ever, like a wonderful erotic love scene.

When I asked my boyfriend if he thinks about me when we make love, he said, 'Oh no, never. I think about having sex with big fat women, or your mother, or my mother . . . ' He gets really sick. It really turns him on to say things like, who'd you fuck this week then? And it really turns him on to hear that I've had sex with other people, people he knows, though he'd go mad if I ever did. But when he's at the height of orgasm he likes me to talk about it. He always brings up black men as well, which is weird, because I've never told him about the black men in my fantasy. He'll say, 'Have you shagged any black men this week?' Sometimes I can come out of it in hysterical laughter; it's funny and an embarrassment. I find it hard to let myself go sometimes. But I always like to think of lots of men doing things to me, soft tongues, and going down on me, bodies with unknown faces.

Caroline aged 24

My situation at the moment is that I'm engaged. I got engaged a year ago, and my fiancé is Italian, and hopefully in about a year's time he'll come over here and we'll get married. It makes life quite difficult, but on the other hand I've got a job here which is quite interesting. I'm just beginning my career and also I want to continue with the research I'm doing, which is in a very specialised field. The company I'm with is just expanding and I'm getting very involved, and it's exciting, so I don't want just to give up the job now and go to Italy and start looking around for work there. My Italian isn't fluent, so it would have been very difficult just to find a job. Eventually we are both hoping to live in Italy, but for me it would be very difficult to start off a career in Italy not being Italian.

So I'm on my own a lot. I fantasise mostly when I'm relaxed. Often I fantasise when I'm on holiday, because I've relaxed and I'm not thinking about others things like work, though I don't think I fantasise that much, or if I do then I'm not all that aware of it. I think the rareness is because I'm rarely actually with my fiancé, so I don't feel very sexy when I'm on my own. When I'm with him or I know I'm going there, or he's coming here, then I can let myself go a bit. I fantasise about him – I don't fantasise about any other specific men.

From very young days I've always had one particular fantasy. I can never really imagine one particular person in that fantasy – it's just a man, he doesn't have an individual face. My father's originally from Sri Lanka, and we used to go and visit my grandfather there. And we always used to go up to bed in the afternoons, for forty winks and to read. I used to sleep in the bed, and the mosquito net would be tied up. It used to hang down from the ceiling and was tied up in the morning after we got up. I'd usually go to bed and read or something, and the mosquito net would be up there, and it used to be very hot and humid, and quite still, and all the windows would be open. The room had windows on three sides, so there used to be a very slight breeze. But it was very hot and humid and sticky, and I used always to have this fantasy about making love to someone in that particular room, underneath the mosquito net when it was

24

opened up over the bed. It's such a strange fantasy to have, and I remember thinking about this when I was still quite young, fourteen, fifteen, sixteen, something like that. I think that the fact that it was very hot and humid and sticky – bodies rubbing against each other getting hotter and sweatier and stickier – is what I found exciting and turned me on.

Quite often I fantasise about how I used to lie in that room, and it's always daytime in my fantasy, when the sun's out and it's hot – the fantasy was never to do with the night-time. We'd be sweating profusely during the day, and we'd cool down at night. I've often thought, what a strange kind of fantasy, and it started when I was so young and still hadn't had any real sexual experiences. I think it could be because the books I used to take upstairs after lunch when we were on holiday usually involved some kind of flirtation, or some kind of romance. I used to take books like *Wuthering Heights*, and books about women who were yearning for men and romance. So the fantasies came because I was reading about these sort of romantic experiences. Often my sister and I – she shared the room and slept in the other bed, next to me – used to just take all our clothes off and lie underneath a cotton bed sheet. I suppose because I was lying there naked under this cotton bedsheet, hot and sticky and reading this very English, prim and proper romance, in my mind I associated those Jane Austen-type yearnings in the books – which never actually mentioned anything about going to bed and sleeping with anyone – with sex. I transformed the romantic glances and things into a different dimension.

Even now that I am much more sexually experienced, I still have that fantasy. Over the summer I went on holiday with my boyfriend to Cyprus. It was very hot and sticky, and I had a field day with my fantasy, which came back so reminiscently in the heat and humidity.

Once when I was at University, I was living in the halls of residence, and I went up with my boyfriend of the time on to the roof. I don't know how we got the idea, but we decided to have a picnic on the roof of the halls of residence, which was a flat roof. So we actually made up a proper picnic hamper, and we went up on to the roof. It was a summer's day, and it was quite nice because there was a lovely view out over Holland Park, and tennis courts and things like that. So we had a really nice picnic up

25

there and then my boyfriend said, 'Come on, let's make love up here.' And I said, 'Are you mad? We're up on the roof!' There were lots of other taller buildings around and so people would probably be able to peer over at us. Eventually we went behind a chimney where it was quite secluded. And I remember the sensation of being out there in the open, being naked and feeling the wind blowing over my naked body, I remember that particular feeling being very exciting, and I think now of similar situations, being outside, nowhere in particular, just being outside and being naked and exposed to all the elements, having them all there. I don't think of the thrill of being out there and that someone might discover you, it's just the natural idea of being outdoors that I find exhilarating and sexually exciting, and fantasise about now.

I remember going for a walk in Richmond Park last autumn and just noticing how deserted it was – it was a weekday in the middle of the day – and it seemed to me to be a really good place to make love. There are plenty of bushes around where you could make love in seclusion, and no one actually comes there. It's a huge park, and it was completely deserted, and in my mind I began to imagine making love there in the open air with the wind blowing softly around me. That's really about as far as the fantasy goes, being naked and outside, no people, plenty of bushes, and a quiet place. Maybe part of the reason I couldn't continue the fantasy was that it was bloody cold! I couldn't possibly actually do something like that at that time of year, it would be far too unpleasant.

My fantasies always tend to revolve round the person I'm with at that time, though occasionally I fantasise about the first time I made love to someone, recalling a past boyfriend. And I love the thrill of the unknown body. I usually can recall very clearly the exact place where that first encounter took place. These fantasies usually happen when I'm thinking about the particular person, not when I've just made love to my fiancé and maybe it hasn't been a particularly earth-moving experience. I drive a lot, and quite often when I'm driving, especially on motorways, I switch off from the driving a bit and start thinking. And, for instance, if I've received a letter from one of my old boyfriends then the fantasy will flash through my mind, his body

26

and how it feels to touch him and explore him. I can usually remember very clearly that feeling of the complete excitement of the first time. In a way this contradicts my ideas about sexual faithfulness, but I will admit to it!

My fantasies tend to be based on things I have done, known experiences taken a bit further. But one thing I'd like to do would be to take my fiancé to that room in Sri Lanka with the bed with the mosquito net above it, and see what would happen. Maybe nothing would happen and it would be the end of my fantasy.

I'm a very faithful person, and I think that that is reflected in my fantasies. I don't fantasise about someone else, because naturally that is how I am. Ever since I knew my fiancé, all the fantasies I've had have always been with him, if anyone at all, though quite often there is no particular identity to the man in my fantasy. I find that's quite interesting. Looking back at the fantasies I've had over the years, it's never other men who I may have met and found physically attractive who feature, and I wouldn't fantasise about that kind of situation or man.

A friend of mine, perhaps more of an acquaintance, once suggested I take part in a group thing with him and another female, three of us. It was the first time that I had thought about it, and I thought it might be quite an interesting thing. Then I went away and thought about it some more, and I couldn't imagine, or fantasise, what it could actually be like. I was keen to try this thing out, just to see how I would react to it, but I just could not fantasise the situation. I knew who the man would be, and we had talked about who the other woman could be, and he'd said he would leave that up to me as I had to be completely comfortable with it, and I sort of had an idea who that other person could be. I tried fantasising the situation, and I had these images in my mind, but they left me cold, they didn't do anything for me. I found the man quite attractive, and perhaps if I'd tried to fantasise about just him and me it would have been a lot easier, but I couldn't picture this thing with three people. And I thought, Well, if I can't even work out the fantasy in my mind, how could I actually play the reality in bed? So I told him I'd give it a miss. It wasn't really me.

27

VIEW FROM THE ARISTOCRACY

View From the Aristocracy

The better off classes in England are well known for their interest in such themes as gardens, clubs and ponies. Here four women of differing ages explain their sexual fantasies. All are well educated and from good families, and their fantasies are perhaps united only by an unusual imagination.

Emma, a slight girl who dabbles in watercolouring, and grew up in a rambling pile on a Northamptonshire Estate, fantasises about taunting stodgy older men at a London Club. When I telephoned her to ask her whether she would participate in my research, she immediately responded, 'Oh no, you're asking the wrong person. I don't like sex much at all.' Clearly she is someone for whom sex has not been of paramount importance, remaining a virgin until she was in her mid-twenties. But she has always been very aware of sexual imagery, and has fantasies about playing games with seduction.

Themes in the minds of Ursula and Sarah revolve around dark foreigners, seduction in the garden, and playing the part of the mistress. Ursula, a diminutive blonde dealer in fine furniture, lives alone in a large old manor house near Henley and in her fantasies tries to relive its history. Her lover has come to Tudor England from the Spanish Court on diplomatic business. In her fantasies, she not only desires and makes love with the stranger, but she is transformed into that period, able to touch the fabrics of their clothes, silk-velvets and lace, and taste the cordials and sweetmeats they drink and eat.

Sarah, quite a shy woman, very slim, with a long mousy pony-tail, does some interior designing, and fantasises about the illicit thrill of being the mistress of a powerful man. 'But I could never kiss and tell to the papers afterwards – the hypocrisy is so sordid.' She lives just outside London in a quiet cottage.

Emily, one of several children, grew up in a central Chelsea house and was mainly brought up by a tough, elderly nanny. Tall and sleek with her Sassoon haircut and small short black skirt, she trained as a beautician and now runs her own business.

Emma aged 35

I have a wonderful fantasy about having sex on the billiard table at a London Club. The Club is a great place to fantasise about because it's always full of lots of stodgy, randy old men and not many young girls; so you get lots of attention and comments, especially if you wear a short skirt. I love to tease.

There are lights above the billiard table, almost like a stage. At the bar I tease the older men whilst actually touching up the younger ones. Only the young ones can have me. I lean on the green expanse of the billiard table with a young man. The men get quite angry, quite indignant that this young man can have possession while the other, prouder, older men are spurned. I'm always followed by a trail of young boys, and spurn the older men. I like that, I like punishing them, watching them calling on their resources to see what they can do to become attractive to me and seduce me. I let them gain a bit of ground, and then drop them in it again. I love deflecting older men, letting them see but not have, displaying myself to them and then having sex in full view with a young whippersnapper. When I go to the Club in reality I find it quite amusing that there is a canopy over the billiard table with a sign on it which reads: 'Members only'.

Sometimes I think of myself as prissy, ethical, a nice girl. I wish that I could really get into contact with the sexual part of me, but I have always found this very difficult. I fantasise about being pure on the one hand and denying myself on the other. I see myself as the forbidden fruit. I was a virgin for a long time, only losing my virginity when I was twenty-five, which was in itself not a confidence-building experience. The man I had sex with, although he was supposed to be a friend, refused to believe that it was my first time. I found this very upsetting – he didn't really know me at all. Ever since losing my virginity I have had nervous breakdowns. Now I fantasise about farm labourers, always the young type with the old farmer intervening, jealous.

I think my earliest fantasy was about being seduced from behind on the library steps. I'm wearing a short skirt and men come up behind me and look up my skirt, then they pull down my knickers and make love to me from behind. Not seeing what's happening as it is all from behind takes away all the responsibility from you.

As an artist, my painting has a kind of sexual parallel; it's a synthesis of my nature. When painting you can no longer argue which part of you is prominent. I get a feeling of complete harmony and unity. When you're painting really really well, it's the equivalent of being able to feel yourself completely but at the same time losing all sense of feeling. You feel really tangible and yet you can't step outside yourself and observe it – it is indescribably but poignant, an ultimate sensation.

What turns me on most is someone really intelligent and witty, so witty that I get left behind. I like the chase, the verbal banter. I once was having a drink in a wine bar with a very clever, witty chap, and we had such a verbal tease – humorous references and other such things – one thing leading on to another, that I had an orgasm just sitting there opposite him. It helps if he is not handsome, as I don't like convention. A secret wit that I don't have access to really turns me on.

My boyfriend is very clever, and I find it quite exciting when he reads to me. I love it that he is so knowledgeable, that he achieves things really quickly, or when he writes letters for me. I find this so attractive that afterwards we immediately go off and make love.

I have a fantasy about a Greek shepherd boy I met when on a painting trip. I was painting in the mountains and I heard a goatherd's bell tinkling along and the shepherd boy came and sat nearish to me outside a church. He plucked a piece of bamboo from a bush and made a flute and then he played a tune.

I fantasise that my boyfriend might have been the shepherd boy. It's the talent, and the fact that he makes the instrument by which he is going to seduce one from scratch that turns me on.

Ursula aged 45

I had a wonderful sexual fantasy, part of which was real, when I went on holiday with a girlfriend. It was a long, long time ago when I was twenty-four, but I have thought about it and elaborated on it over the years. We went to Mauritius, and stayed in a wonderful hotel where they had little chalets on the beach. The second day we were there we walked on to the beach to do some swimming, and there was a very beautiful Mauritian selling silks. We went to the stall and he draped a lot of different silks – they were saris mostly – on me, and I bought two. And then because we were there I met him every day and he asked me out. He was making a lot of money for that sort of island, and so he took me to some wonderful restaurants and we had a fabulous affair. But it was all so sexual because he was dark, and very beautiful, and totally un-Western. He'd go swimming and dive for lobsters, then we'd have a barbecue on the beach and he'd drape me in silks, and it was all very exciting. Lots of sex, rolling about on the warm beach at night, under the stars.

I love to fantasise about that affair because it was all so tied up with a beautiful country, fabulous silks to wear, gorgeous restaurants to visit and all that lying around on the beach making love. And he was so unfucked up by any sort of Western values. Like the noble savage. The sex was so wonderful and natural. He was like Tarzan – he had this wonderful coloured skin, glorious glossy black hair, and lovely bone structure, and he was tall and had a great body – and he touched and held and caressed me so confidently. He treated me like a queen. I wasn't expecting to meet anybody, and there he was. He swam well, he hunted, he collected shells and sold them. He was so physical, and clever enough to make money out of just natural things.

Sometimes I have a sort of romantic *Frenchman's Creek* fantasy about the river at the bottom of my garden. I imagine being swept away amongst the flowers in my garden, particularly when the Regale Lilies are in full bloom, because the scent is intoxicating, and they come out at the time when the roses and the honeysuckle are out. It's a scented garden, a garden for all the senses.

Therefore it would be very nice if somebody, a troubadour or some Tudor man, came down by barge and climbed over the wall. He would take me into the gazebo and we would make love. I'd be wearing luscious clothes, lovely silks, and negligés and silk-velvet, very sensuous. He'd be a dark foreigner come over from something like the Spanish Court on diplomatic business in Tudor England, and he'd be wearing black velvet and be bejewelled, and be from an extremely good family. I'd serve him sweetmeats and cordials and then I'd get thrown on the bed and slowly seduced. He undresses me slowly but urgently, full of desire and passion. Layer upon layer of my beautiful clothes are cascading to the floor. We make love in several different positions and for a very long time, breaking to eat more sweetmeats and drink more cordials, and to bathe in rose-water. He makes me feel gorgeous and passionate, my body like the smooth silks and delicate lace I am wearing. We seem to glide into different positions with little sweat and effort, his deep thrusts penetrating my whole body. He gets orgasm after orgasm and still stays stiff for more and more.

I like the man to take control in bed. In a way, I'm the boring one, slightly passive in bed, involved but not aggressive, not calling all the shots. I much prefer to be taken than to take. I'm very bad if a man doesn't know about his own sexuality because I can't play that slightly more masculine role. I'm hopeless at it because I don't have the self-confidence, or the inclination. I like the man to be the knowledgeable one, to take what he wants and give pleasure in return.

I love the idea of being seduced by a dark foreigner. Being seduced and made love to by a wolf, like in the Angela Carter story, *Company Of Wolves*, would be my ultimate fantasy. I have the film on video and watch it often as it makes me very excited and turned on. It's about werewolves – men who turn into wolves.

The heroine goes into the woods on the way to her grandmother's – it's the Red Riding Hood story. On the way she meets a foreign traveller, a man, and he's got eyebrows that meet in the middle. It all takes place in the nineteenth century, so he's wearing velvet trousers and a lacy shirt and black velvet jacket. She has her basket, a picnic, with her, and they sit down to eat the picnic, then they have a bet as to who can get to the grandmother's house first: her if she follows the path, and him if he goes through the wood, because he knows the area very well. He arrives first at the grandmother's house and breaks down the door, then goes in and kills the grandmother. She arrives and he is there waiting for her, and he seduces her, makes love to her savagely and violently. He is really a wolf and gradually turns into one, the wolf coming out almost like flesh from within. And she, because he has made love to her and probably impregnated her with some sort of animal physiognomy, also begins to change. So they both turn into wolves and jump out of the house with a great leap, smashing through a plate-glass window, to live together.

I find wolves a turn-on, not dogs, but wolves, because they are so dark, dangerous, unknown. I find that a turn-on, being licked all over by that harsh and dangerous tongue. Not that I want to buy an alsatian dog and make love with it! But wolves are humanised in stories, turning back and forth into men and wolves. I fantasise about the idea of having a lover who is a wolf as well as a man. A dark fantasy, tinged with something slightly sinister. The wood is wonderful in the film and in my mind – lots of creepy-crawlies, and the light between the trees in the forest is fascinating, drawing you into a darker world where these mysterious things go on.

There's also a wedding party where a girl has been wronged, a girl from the village who is pregnant. She comes into the marquee where the man who has made her pregnant is actually in the process of getting married to somebody of his own social class, and she humiliates them, then turns the whole of the wedding party into wolves. The whole thing happens in slow motion. It's clever and it's slightly decadent in a sexual way. I like opulent, sinister decadence and degeneracy.

Sarah aged 28

Sex was something that was quite hidden in the family I came from. My parents divorced when I was ten, and even though there was this turmoil going on I had no idea at all what it was about. It all got very confusing when I was in my teens. I didn't really think about sex at all until I went to college. I was a virgin until I was twenty-one, I'm twenty-eight now. It was important to me to stay a virgin. My whole life was controlled by other people and that was the only way I could control myself.

I had four brothers, one a stepbrother, and a sister. They were all away at school, so we didn't really know what they were getting up to. It turns out that they got up to quite extraordinary things. My brother is gay. I didn't know; he knew when he was fourteen. I had crushes on people at that stage and that was about it. I was more interested in ponies. I used to fancy my brother's friend. We used to go jogging together after school, and I used to fantasise about being tackled to the ground. I must have been about sixteen. I think he once gave me a lovebite, but that was about it.

I felt very pressured into my first full sexual experience because all my friends were very sexually active around me. I think that because my parents were in such turmoil, it was important to me to be in control of the situation, though I can't say I was very careful about choosing the person. He was very insignificant, really; it was very disappointing.

Somewhere along the line I developed an attraction for older men. Perhaps it was to find a father figure, but more probably because we had some very dishy teachers at school. We all used to fantasise about our teachers, and we each had a particular teacher that we fantasised about. There were four or five men in their mid-twenties who lived in the same house. I didn't board, I was a daygirl, but there was just this incredible house with all these dishy young men in it teaching us. We knew that they'd go out with girls in the sixth form, and we all used to sit around and fantasise about what each one had done. Mine was the Drama teacher. It was a very basic fantasy, flirtations and being chatted up, mainly. I think to this day I still feel quite repressed sexually, and I still find it quite difficult to talk about. I won't get involved

38

with someone unless I really care about them. Even when it comes to fantasies, I probably wouldn't go that far.

I'm in a bit of a strange situation now, because I've been seeing a married man for about six years and he's my constant sexual fantasy really, and occasionally the fantasies come true. All my sexual thoughts are channelled his way. It's very frustrating, but it's nice sometimes. They're never outrageous – fantasies are things that could come true, and they do occasionally. My fantasies are incredibly boring domestic fantasies. I'll cook for him and then we'll go to bed, or have a bath together – just normal things that aren't the same with my boyfriend, because it's naughty and his unavailability gives it the edge, which is quite nice.

When I first met this man six years ago I lived with him for a year and a half, so we have had that background to our relationship, but the longer I know him the more it fades away. I think he fantasises about me, but who can guess what men fantasise about? I'm sure it's all rather basic. But now I've done things recently like stay the odd night in a hotel with him, which is quite a nice fantasy situation. Most of my fantasies tend to be reliving things we've done together.

I was at a petrol station the other day and this huge Mercedes swept in beside me and this incredibly tall man (I've got a thing about tall men because they're so protective) came in and went in front of me at the station. I thought, if I had a business card or something on me now I'd give it to him, he was so gorgeous. He was probably about fifty, but had a real boy's face and lovely twinkly blue eyes and really brown skin, and I looked into his car, and there was his frumpy wife sitting there with his teenage daughter. And he was the ideal person to have an affair with. Just a brief fantasy, but very much my kind of thing.

I'd like to have a card printed with 'Rent a Mistress'. I find it quite exciting and risqué to be the other woman. I've always fantasised about having an affair with a politician. It would be so exciting, but I could never kiss and tell to the papers afterwards – the hypocrisy is so sordid. The man that I do see is probably as near to a politician as I'll ever get, a boring businessman, but he works in the City and wears a suit. My whole world, a creative one, is so alien to that, that I find the City irresistible.

39

I think that in fantasies there should, to some extent, be an element of things coming true. In a way I can't fantasise because I'm already in a fantasy situation. You're constantly waiting for opportunities to do illicit things. You get used to it, but it's not normal, and it makes having any normal sort of relationship seem very boring and dull. Maybe that's why I get so bored with boyfriends if I see them every night. Often my relationship with the married man can get very dull as well. I can feel just like a second wife to him – he's not the most romantic of men. But I probably think about him several times every day, and that's really a fantasy, because I know that he'll never be mine.

His wife has moved back in, and we don't have sex very often. That's probably why I spend so much more time fantasising. I fantasise to the extent that when I'm sleeping with another boyfriend I'll always think about him. That's the only way I can make it bearable at the moment, through fantasy. I just dread that any relationship I might have is going to be like that, though perhaps if I had the man I want I'd get bored with him and move on to someone else. So perhaps my fantasy is to be a mistress figure. To a certain extent it makes you very independent. And I'm very independent.

Emily aged 27

What I wonder when I think about sexual fantasy is whether other people think about the same things as me. I've never really discussed it with anyone.

I have several fantasies and I think I interchange them, and they change over the years. It's not something that's static, it's something that develops. My fantasy takes place at several different places. I'm waiting at a table or something, and someone puts their fingers up my legs and goes into my vagina and then – normally I'm forced into this situation, so I'm not responsible, I'm being forced into it – I'm forced to sit on their penis under the table. I'm sitting beside the table, and they're underneath, obscured from view.

It's always in a public place, a restaurant or pub, or it could be at an executive meeting, or it could be in my surgery. It's nobody in particular doing this to me, just anybody, a blob! I've never really thought about what they look like, it's just the feeling of powerlessness. Sometimes it varies, and I'm a child being punished for doing something bad and it's a headmaster or authority figure of some sort, but that's different, I'm not my own age.

I've often wondered whether this was a very immature version of the fantasy. And I have tried to remember what fantasies I had when I was younger and where I got the original idea for my main fantasy from. I think I started having these fantasies through reading literature, books that my brothers used to have around the house. Not romantic books. My brothers used to have very rude, slightly pornographic novels – nothing terribly serious, but lewd enough to give me quite a thrill. I'm not sure what I would have done if I hadn't had brothers!

My fantasy does vary, it's never static. Where I am in the fantasy often changes, and how many people are around, and how I'm forced into the situation.

On reflection, I think it's the form of penetration that excites me most, rather than just the situation. It's the idea of the man sitting down and me being forced straight on to him, because that never varies; rather than the place we're in, which does vary.

I'm not sure how this relates to my actual life. I've never had

41

secretive relationships. Most of my sexual learning experience wasn't done with my husband, so I tend to hark back to previous experience. My husband isn't particularly flexible in the ways that he'd have sex, and previous relationships were more flexible, so I expect that's probably why my fantasies hark back to that period. Now it's all more conservative, less imagination. In fact I actually tend to fantasise when we're actually making love, which is a bit sad really. I don't remember doing that years ago. I asked my husband whether he fantasised as well, but he wouldn't tell me. I think often one person in a relationship is more open than the other. It's not as if you actually want to have sex with anyone else – fantasy is all in the imagination, another level.

I enjoy elaborating on my basic fantasy. I can actually be at the office, answering the phone and doing other work whilst I'm being forced into having sex in my fantasy. I have a funny idea that I would like to live the fantasy. But I wouldn't like it at all if I found myself actually in any of the situations; it would be completely horrible. I hate being out of control. I don't know why I should fantasise about being forced into something. Maybe it's because I've never really been forced into it. Maybe that is the element of sexual excitement: doing something that I would never do, and the element of danger and fear. I've never really thought of that element of force before, but it was always there.

In this modern world, I'm not terribly liberated. In fact I'm quite old-fashioned. My fantasies are about having the responsibility taken out of my hands. I'm quite narrow, and I've not had an awful lot of experiences. I had a sheltered upbringing, a sheltered life. When I do my counselling for Cruise, there are many things that shook me: alcoholism, drugs, and the relationships that people have with them. That's quite an eye-opener – it makes me realise just how little I know about people, and people's lives. So I am very square. On the other hand, I'm a woman in my twenties with my own career and own business, and there's a degree of liberation in that. But still I'm in a formal relationship and have been for a long time, and have no intention of having a relationship on the side, which is pretty square.

At first I thought that my fantasies were completely separate from each other, but then when I looked at them I could see that they weren't. It was all the same area of fantasy. I'm sure that the fantasy has changed as I've changed, especially in the location of the fantasy, which has changed according to what I'm doing in my life. I always fantasise about definite physical places. Apart from being caught in this potentially compromising situation at work or in a restaurant, my fantasy isn't terribly detailed. Sometimes I'm the waitress in the restaurant and the man calls me over and he says, 'Don't move from this position,' and then he puts his fingers up me and then he makes me sit on his cock, and that's about it really. It doesn't go any further, it just stops at that point. I just relive that whole stage over and over again, I don't get any further.

THE ARTS

The Arts

The women who discuss their sexual background and fantasies in this section are all involved in the arts, in a variety of different ways – such as textile art, acting, sculpting and photography.

Michelle, a thirty-nine-year-old sculptress, has recently come out of a long and sexually depressing relationship and begun to discover her sexual self. A very physical person, her fantasies used to be about her large motherly figure enveloping her lover. Now she has lost weight and her fantasies are beginning to be about taking sexually as well as giving. Tall and strikingly elegant it was hard to imagine her not attracting many lovers.

Carol, now a landscape photographer, imagines she is dancing with her lover and is seduced by the rhythm and the music. Both Tina, a rotund, ash-blonde artist who designs textiles and is both passionate and experimental in the large bright pieces she creates, and Harriet, a flamboyant actress who works as a temp between acting jobs, like to act out their fantasies, both for their lovers' and for their own benefits, enjoying experimentation.

All four women I have included here come from backgrounds that were not at all open sexually. They appear to have channelled their repressed sexual energy into creative pursuits. In addition to this they have each built up an area in their lives of complex and detailed sexual fantasies.

Michelle aged 39

Sex was never mentioned at all at home when I was growing up. The only time I realised that my parents actually had sex was when we moved house to a bigger city. I realised they were actually doing things on a Friday night because everything would go quiet – they'd stop shouting at each other. There was no demonstration of sex at all in our house – no holding hands, or arms around each other, or anything like that. It was definitely very repressed. Church was a big part of our lives. I can remember vividly some friends of the family who, when sex was mentioned in the church one Sunday, left and never came back. It was very much taboo.

I had sexual fantasies as a child, five or six years old. I've thought about them again recently. They were about things like men pissing on me. I often wonder if it was somehow to do with my older brother. He was ten when I was a baby, and he liked to look after me. He used to want to take the baby to bed. Maybe he was still taking me to bed as a two-year-old, and maybe he was still doing things to me, because where on earth as a five-year-old did I get the idea of men pissing on me if there was nothing to relate it to at all? If sex is completely repressed, where on earth does all that come from? I still wonder whether my brother was doing something or not.

We moved around a lot for one reason or another, as my father changed jobs. I remember one place we went to live where I used to have this thing about dressing up. I used to go out into the country in the height of summer, and I'd get dressed up with all these groundsheets and greatcoats of my father's around me. And I'd be fantasising about a man keeping me in that situation. I'd either be really hot, and someone would be keeping me extremely hot, or I'd be very cold and someone would be making me take all my clothes off. That was when I was about seven. It was very exciting. I used to go out with the intention of playing this fantasy through in one way or another.

At that time we rented a house right out in the country, from when I was about seven to about the age of ten. It was a big house with large windows, and my window didn't have any curtains. It was quite a distance from the road, along which very little traffic came, but yet I can remember that I used to stand up there against the window, naked, imagining that men driving past would be able to see me. And I used to fantasise about that a lot.

We move around a lot and life changed. We moved from the depths of the countryside into a remote town and then into the city, and my ideas changed. Because of peer pressures I wanted to be accepted. At that time, the late sixties, early seventies, everything was happening, but sometimes a good fantasy was just a good snog, quite basic. The idea of being wanted, desired, was what I needed. I don't think there were many more fantasies than that during my teenage years. It was just about exploring sex really.

One fantasy that I have had since then is about big tits. I used to be a lot fatter than I am now, and then I had big tits. The fantasy was that I'd be happily married to someone and we'd really be in love, and my ideal sexual fantasy would then be that I'd be fucking this man and I'd have a baby on each tit as well. I don't know what it's really like – I don't have children – but that's something that always's been in the back of my mind, a major thing. I've lots a lot of weight recently, and that whole fantasy has taken a step back. Tits were a big thing before, and now they're not so much. It's strange, a few stone has made a big difference to the way I feel about myself. I was quite proud of my tits, they were big things in a way, and that was a big fantasy; and now that they're no longer big it's no longer a big fantasy. I think the fantasy had something to do with my idea of the perfect family, in the sense that you could be doing everything – you could be a mother and a lover, everything at the same time, and everyone's involved in it.

I've changed everything about myself now that I'm slimmer. The way that I dress, for instance, little skirts. My whole life has changed recently. I was with someone for nine years and basically he wasn't interested in me sexually. I turned off completely then. It was like you just switch the whole thing off, you couldn't even deal with fantasies in a way, it was just too much. If someone's not interested in you and you're with them, it's too much for your mind, so you turn off the whole sexual thing completely. The first sexual experience I had after that time, which woke me up and changed everything around me, was quite freaky. I couldn't sit still for days. I just wanted dicks inside me all the time, it was awful. I wanted so much sex because I had kept this thing repressed inside me for such a long time, so the first experience I had after that made me hot all the time. I wanted anything and everything. I couldn't stop thinking and fantasising about fucking, having big dicks inside me all the time. When you're having sex you even repress the fantasies, because it's so hurtful being treated like that, that you hold back everything. Now it's all turned back on again over the last six months.

I lost all that weight very quickly, several stone in about a month. I didn't mean to, I think it was just the stress of being out of one long-term miserable relationship and into such an exciting one. I just thought that if I ate I'd throw up, it was really strange. Now I fantasise in different ways. The fantasies are more to do with my lover, definitely about him. He's quite into the fantasies as well. He's black, and when we're having sex he'll say things like, 'You've got this big black dick inside you.' At first I made a bit of a joke about it and said why does it have to be black, it's you, and that sort of thing, but then I do find that it is quite a powerful image in a way – mainly because you're lying there in bed with someone and, though I don't think my skin's particularly white, you can look down and the contrast is so beautiful. That's amazing really, and that does turn me on.

I think he's quite sexually powerful. He's helped me so much, having spent nine years with somebody who didn't really want me at all. That was a weird relationship, with someone who wants you, but they want you as a mother rather than as someone they can have a proper sexual relationship with. Then to meet this man who is quite powerful sexually is just wonderful. I still fantasise now that I'm with him, but it's more to do with reliving sexual experiences we've had together, and more to do with having a loving relationship with someone rather than just the sexual thing. Though I do still fantasise about sex, it's more of a quiet thing now. Having said that, now that everything's changed for me, and my whole personality has opened up, just about anything turns me on! Men turn me on and even seeing beautiful women can turn me on as well.

Being a sculptress, I find anything that's beautiful exciting. I think that the best sculptures have got an element of sexuality in them. There is sexuality in most good art, and that's what makes it powerful in a way, even when it's understated. When you're working as a sculptress and you've got your hands in the clay, you forget about everything you're doing, in a sense. It's all coming out then. Your own kind of sensuality, the power and the energy of your sexuality, all comes through and is portrayed in your work.

I don't know if my work has changed since I've changed. Lots of work I used to do during that period of repression was really sexual. I wonder now whether, having in a sense been freed, it would come through in my work again, or whether there is no longer any need for it to come through so dominantly in my work again.

Carol aged 45

Sex was never talked about in my family, oh no, goodness me!

I went to art school, and when you go to art school you discover sex in a very, very good way. Art school in the sixties was a very big thing, very moody; you all wore black and had white make-up, black eyes. You do everything that everybody else doesn't do, you make a point of it. Some of the students actually lived together, which was not happening then at all, a major event. It was all quite shocking compare to my parents' view, but I thought it was just wonderful, all these people dressing in very odd clothes, doing things that nobody else had done.

The art students influenced me a lot because before that I was brought up in a religious family with heavy morals: don't do this, don't do that. When I got to art school I suddenly discovered that there was another life outside the small Norfolk village I came from.

I hitch-hiked to London a lot. I met this guy in a pub called the Duke of somewhere. He was a hippy and he was wonderful looking, a bit like a gypsy with black hair, and I had an affair with him. He was the first person that I slept with. That was really weird because he invited me to his house, and his parents were school teachers, really strict people, and I lost my virginity on the carpet by the stairs with them sleeping upstairs. I remember thinking, Is this it?

As art students then we thought we were the bee's knees. We were ten years ahead, and I was heavily influenced by being there. At that stage I was too busy doing it and experimenting to fantasise much. At that time sex wasn't very much in the open, so we were doing it and thinking that everybody else wasn't. Art students were allowed to do it because we were considered to be strange people, whereas other people weren't. My mother strongly disapproved. If I hadn't gone to art school I wouldn't have done it, because of the village and my parents and the whole bit.

The art students gave me the courage to have boyfriends, sex, go to London, be what I thought was outrageous. I love to be outrageous. In my imagination it was exciting to do outrageous things that I'd been taught not to do. That's what turned me on, that and the disapproval.

I had fantasies about doing outrageous things, probably because I had such a strict upbringing. It was heavily religious – we had to go to church every Sunday, we had to go to Sunday School and do all of that. Nothing was ever discussed. Even when I had my period, it was a surprise to me and everybody else; nobody told me about it. I was a rebel. I met a black man twenty years older than myself when I was only seventeen, and was very impressed with his life. By the time I was eighteen we had a child. I was doing everything I was brought up not to do, and I've never looked back.

I've always in a way done my fantasy, which was to rebel and have affairs with unlikely men. I continue to do that. I've always found it sexually exciting to be different, with a black man or anyone my mother would disapprove of. With him it was curiosity as well, and going against the grain, because most nice white girls from my village married a nice white boy from next door and got on with it, so I didn't.

I found the black man exciting because he was a different colour, a different age, and he was very sophisticated, which I wasn't. I was from a country village with grass growing out of my head. I think he taught me a lot sexually because he was older than me, more experienced. He played music in a club, and I used to go down there in my little dress and dance.

Now I'm on my own, my man is in prison, and I'm left with my fantasies. I fantasise about hunky black guys mostly. I never really fantasise about the prison, but the visiting room can be a very sexually charged place – not only on a fantasy level, because I've actually seen women do it in the visiting room. They sit on his knee wearing a skirt, and then lever themselves up and on to his cock. I could never do that – a complete embarrassment, I couldn't ever get it together – but I've seen it. The visiting room is a very large room with teeny tables. You sit on two sides next to each other, then she moves her chair round to the corner and slides on to his lap.

The most erotic thing for me is dancing. A guy that can dance to me is very sexy. Recently when in wales I met a very pretty twenty-five-year-old, one of those people who's there, in a club, and won't go away, but he could dance, and if a man can dance I'm gone. Most English men can't dance, and this man could really dance, and I thought yes, I'm there. That's the most sexy thing that can happen to me, being with a man that can dance. For me it's the music and the man combined; he is moving his hips and his shoulders to wonderful music. This man was really wonderful. I have been thinking about him and this situation ever since. He was doing a sort of courting dance goading me into joining him, and with the dancing, his hips, the movement, the atmosphere, I was drawn to him, to join in. In my mind this scene becomes sexual and there is nobody there but us caught in slow, sensual dance, the rhythm, the hot sweating bodies. I can feel my whole body moving towards him and being drawn in to become part of him. On the dance floor I am transported into another world, hot, sensual, passionate; and when we make love it is part of the dance and the music.

Tina aged 38

My home background was not very progressive or open sexually. In fact, I never saw my father naked in my whole life, or even in his underwear. If he wasn't fully dressed, he always wore a dressing gown. There was never any talk of sex. They didn't tell me anything until I was nine years old and I was given a book to read. I suppose it could have been because my parents were older parents – my father was forty-six when I was born, and came from a very uptight family, and my mother was thirty-six. I don't think they ever talked to us about sex, only in terms of how babies come into the world, but nothing beyond a very basic explanation with the book.

I had some very, very early experiences of sexual fantasy. When I was about four or five one of the kids in the neighbourhood came into kindergarten all excited. We had a character locally who'd had polio when he was younger, he must have been about ten years older than us. We thought he was very big and frightening, he limped and he was always very nasty and aggressive to everybody. And this girl said, 'You know what, you know what, I saw him in the basement of our house, and he was sitting on a chair and there was this woman who was naked, and I couldn't see who she was because she had her back to me, and she was sucking his cock.'

This was a revelation to me, because from then on I thought that that's how people had sex, because I had no idea. So all my fantasies were oral ones, because I thought that the way people had sex was that the women went down and sucked the man's cock. That was my idea of how things went. I used to have all these fantasies about that, and it took me a long time to realise that this wasn't actually the way it was done. Even when I read this book about how children come into the world it didn't connect to sex; this was reproduction, and that was sex. That was much more erotic for me than the book. The book had diagrams and Mummy explained it to me, and there was nothing erotic at all in the book, just mummies and daddies and babies and hospitals, like a story. But my fantasy was to do with peeking through a window and seeing something you shouldn't see, it was to do with sexual organs, so that image became my fantasy.

When I was about six we started school. There was a boy about three years older than I was and I thought he was gorgeous and I really had a crush on him. I used to have a fantasy that they took all the school tables into the yard and put them in rows, and all the boys had to take their trousers off and lie there just in their underpants. Then each girl had to pick a number or a name out of a hat, sometimes it was a number and sometimes it was a name. They had to go to the table where the boy they'd selected was lying, or the table that was marked with the number, and suck the boy's penis, and I of course always got the table with the boy I liked. It was wonderful. That was my earliest sexual fantasy. Psychologically perhaps my early sexual thoughts just fell into the oral stage.

After that I began to play 'doctors and nurses' with the other children, and that sort of thing. I suppose that this was quite a bit later. I had two neighbours that I used to play with. One of them did in fact become a doctor, I met him recently! I used to go over to play at his house in the afternoon when my parents were resting. You could make a noise at his house because there were no parents resting – his were out at work. I was always the patient and the other little girl was always the nurse and the boy was always the doctor. We used to play all sorts of games. They always used to have to examine me down below and check everything, and so on. And this became my great fantasy, him being a doctor and checking me over.

I can't remember having any fantasies for a whole period after that, just a sort of numbness for a while before I got to puberty. When I got to puberty it was all boyfriends and girl-friends, things were beginning to happen sexually and I understood more about it all. Hormonally there were things happening, so my experiences tied in with that. But I didn't have much in the way of fantasies except for romantic ones – going out with somebody, having my first kiss. I used to think about being a couple, holding hands and writing notes to each other at school, going to a film together, and what it would be like if my parents went away for the weekend and we had the house to ourselves. The fantasies were more about what it would be like to be a couple rather than sexual fantasies.

Quite early on I had a boyfriend for a long time and then I

actually started having proper sex, not just playing around. After a few months I started fantasising about what it would be like with other men because I'd had no proper sexual experience with anyone else. At first it had been terribly exciting with the boyfriend because we were discovering different ways and feelings, but then I started wondering what it would be like with somebody else. Not that I wasn't happy with my boyfriend, it was just a kind of natural curiosity – is it going to be the same? Is it going to be different? So I went and did it with two other people just to find out, and it ruined the relationship.

Had I been older I might have told him about my feelings and we could have fantasised about it together, but I didn't, and being young I just had to go and do it, and he was hurt and didn't understand and that was the end of the relationship. He was fantasising about getting married and setting up home together, walking past furniture shops saying don't you like that settee and isn't that a lovely carpet, and I was fantasising about what it would be like to sleep with other men, so we weren't at the same point in our lives at all. The more he fantasised about furniture the more oppressed I felt. I needed to go out and experiment.

At about the age of eighteen I used to fantasise over the weekend papers. At the time there were a lot of stories about free love and things like Scandinavian sex shows and sex shops. Everything was going on at that time, and the papers were reporting it. I used to fantasise about being part of that world. Things like being in a live sex show – with my boyfriend, of course. People would be looking at us. I was young then and thought we were very beautiful, and our bodies looked very beautiful. The fantasy was about living in a world outside the world I was in, which would make me much freer.

I felt very provincial. Living in a provincial town there was a feeling that everybody knew your business, and that people were gossiping behind your back, and if you slept with too many men you got nicknamed and looked at. So I felt that the exciting sex world was a world I couldn't be part of because of social circumstances.

My father died when I was a teenager, and that actually liberated me a lot, because he was very, very strict about having sex before marriage, and having sex before I was twenty-one. He

57

made me make all sorts of promises, and I used to feel very guilty about having sex at the beginning. But after he died I felt like I was going on a revenge trip. He made me make all these promises and then he died. So I thought, screw him, I'm going to do exactly what I want to do, and in a way it was a very freeing experience. My mother couldn't cope with all this, so she took me to the doctor and put me on the pill, and said, 'Go ahead, do whatever you want as long as you don't get pregnant.'

At first as an art student I lived on a houseboat in Hammersmith with a director of children's television programmes and an ex-nun who was learning to be a probation officer. I began to feel very inadequate because he was much older than me – he seemed terribly grown up at the time – and he worked for television. So I began to use my fantasies in order to enhance my sex life, so I could pretend to be more experienced than I actually was, and to live up to what I thought his expectations were. I felt like I was little again, which was strange, because I had begun to feel grown up with all the sexual activity. I fantasised about being glamorous and desired, and dressing in all sorts of fancy clothes and performing for him. The funny thing was that he kept telling me about his previous girlfriend, who became completely frigid over the years. He loved her dearly, but the reason they broke up was that they didn't have a sex life any more. So in a way, on the one hand I felt that there was a one-upmanship there, but on the other hand I felt very dirty because I was very sexual at the time. He'd been with this person who he felt a sort of platonic love for, because there was no sex, and also we were living with this nun, so I thought maybe I ought to be a Holy Madonna type. I used to dress very prim and proper on the outside, an then at night when we got into bed I would switch roles in my head. It was like acting all the time.

After that I got into a very weird scene sexually, and I think I stopped fantasising because I was actually doing so many strange things. Since then I've had no need to fantasise about being in threesomes and foursomes because I did it so often.

Now, as an adult, when I have a permanent partner, once the relationship stabilises I tend to share my fantasies with them – not necessarily to act them out, because it's not always possible to act them out, but we say what they are, and it's actually a turn-on to voice them in bed. This is different to fantasising on your own, because there's actually somebody there, and the fantasy grows into a sort of ritual, a habit fantasy.

The main fantasy is an exhibitionist one of someone watching, then later on joining in. Somebody comes in by accident and sees us making love and then gets undressed and joins in. It's not necessarily somebody I know, or somebody I know well – it could be just somebody I've casually seen on the street or fancied at a party, or a friend of my husband's whom I have no intention of going to bed with in real life – but it is a way of doing it without betraying the relationship. I think instead of doing what I did when I was younger, of being curious about somebody else and going out and doing it, what I did was bring the person into bed in fantasy. Gradually I have been able to say these things and then my husband was able to say things to me, like he would pick up some teenager school girl and bring her home in his fantasy and we would fantasise how we would all three of us make love together. Because it was a fantasy and it was shared it wasn't threatening at all; it was sexually enhancing to the relationship.

Another thing I used to fantasise about was standing in a bus or public place and somebody coming up behind me, and not being able to see who they were, and just feeling him lift my skirt and start making love to me in the middle of a crowd, or feel him rubbing against me. And then when I got off the bus I'd hear footsteps behind me and know that any minute now I was going to get to a dead end in the road and then it was going to happen. The excitement of not knowing who it was, and knowing that the footsteps were leading to something, was very sexual.

Some of my past fantasies have ceased to be fantasies now because I acted them out. I used to have fantasies about bondage, and then I got into a relationship with a man who was really into it. After we'd acted it out for so many months it just became a part of my life, and it wasn't a fantasy any more. One thing I never fantasise about is somebody causing me pain. I don't find the idea of pain at all arousing. But I used to find the idea of being overpowered very relaxing, not having to do anything. I like the idea of just being there and somebody else enjoying me sexually and causing me pleasure without me having to do anything. I tend to take a lot of responsibility within a relationship,

59

so I think the fantasy of having somebody else take responsibility for me and for my pleasure, and being totally passive in a relationship, was very arousing for me. That's why I wanted to act it out, to know how it would actually feel in real life. Having acted it ut, I find I don't fantasise about that any more. I've lived through it, it's gone.

Before I had children I used to fantasise that I was a school teacher seducing young school boys, telling them to stay on after class, and making love to them sitting on their teacher's desk. They would be boys in their first stage of puberty, twelve- and thirteen-year-olds, in shorts, I'd be seducing them, instructing them to take off their clothes, and locking the classroom, sitting on the teacher's desk making love to them, or going up to the boy's loo and locking them in one of the cubicles and making love to them there. There would be the risk of losing my job and all the tension of that, and on the other hand they'd never done it before, so it was the first time and very exciting. Since I've had kids I can't fantasise about that any more, because it could have been somebody doing it to my child. Suddenly it seems like child abuse.

Some of my fantasies are too dangerous to want to do, like having a total stranger come up behind you in a bus – I wouldn't live that fantasy out. But some things you can live out if you have a partner you can trust. I remember one hysterical case of trying to live out a partner's fantasy. He was older, and he had a fantasy about seducing a school girl, which I think many men have. So there was me, big woman that I am, dressed in a tiny little red skirt, and little white socks, and little ballerina shoes. I had to go out of the room and knock on the door, and he was lying on the bed reading the paper with his pants open, saying come in little girl what do you want. And I had to go along with this, but in the middle I just burst out laughing, because it was never my fantasy, and I just couldn't relate to it. He was terribly offended. It was just one of those things, you can't always get into somebody else's fantasy. I really tried and I played the part and I dressed up, and I tried to understand it, but suddenly looking at myself, big me in this tiny little red skirt, I just couldn't do it. It was so funny that there was nothing sexual about it. He shouted at me to go out and do it again, which I did, but I exploded with laughter again at the same point and this time he joined in the laughter, and we never tried that one again. Sometimes trying to turn fantasies into reality just doesn't work.

My current fantasies are very much affected by my divorce and separation from my husband after many years. Up to a few months after the split, no matter who I tried to fantasise about, I always saw his face and his hands and him being there, and there was something very upsetting about it, because of course he wasn't there. It became very difficult to have a nice, pure, wholesome sexual fantasy because this sense of bereavement and loss kept coming into it. It took me quite a while, until I was actually able to go to bed with someone else after a year or so, to release myself from this fantasy.

Now I find it easier, and I can fantasise about men I've been to bed with in the past and recent lovers. Basically they all have faces in my fantasies, and I used the fantasy life to relive past sexual experiences, much more so than in the past, when I used fantasies to try out things that I couldn't actually do in reality. Now I find myself wanting to relive things from the past. Now I'm not thinking about exciting new things, but focusing on something I feel safe with that's familiar. It gives a sense of security, because I'm on my own, to fantasise about people I've been with and I know I've had good sex with. Sometimes I take it to more of an extreme, things I actually did with them, but they have names and faces and are very definite people rather than strangers off the street. It's because of the change in my status. I don't want to fantasise about some man coming in off the street, which is threatening and dangerous, whereas I would have done from the security of my married life.

At the moment sexual fantasy is very important to me. I think the more active I was sexually the less the fantasies played a role, and I find now that they play a far greater role than they have done in recent adult life, because I don't have a partner and I don't have an active sex life. So in between I fantasise about having a sex life. I feel it keeps me in touch with my sexual feelings rather than stagnating or getting into a sense of loneliness. Also there's a certain element of release of tension, of being able to get out of where you are now and be somewhere else, and also express a certain longing, which I think is a healthy longing, to have a sex life again.

Fantasies keep us alive in a sexual way even if we're on our own. They keep me in touch and alive. My fantasies are very explicit, and they actually go through all the stages, from foreplay to making love, to coming. In a way there is something very relieving about it, that I am still alive sexually. For a year after the end of my marriage I hardly had a sex life, but at least in my fantasy world it continued. And in the fantasy world I was clinging to images that were secure and comforting and felt good to me rather than going for strangers without faces, because I think at the moment all my future sexual partners are strangers without faces. I think it's very interesting how fantasy has evolved through age, experience, social conduct, puberty, all sorts of things. There are clearly different stages of fantasy which with me are affected by how sexually active I am, and if I had the sort of partner I could share fantasies with, I would.

Harriet aged 40

The fantasy that I use the most is something that I have now been able to pass on to my boyfriend as well. I'm very turned on by the idea of doing something sexual, firstly with the risk of being caught, and then actually in a public place so that people do catch us.

Originally I used to set up a scenario for myself. I would pretend I was in an office, in a high-powered position, and I would be conducting an interview with somebody, perhaps somebody who was applying for a job, and while I was conducting the interview an invisible hand would come up and masturbate me. The thing that gave the fantasy its greatest excitement was the idea of trying to conduct the interview without giving away to the interviewee what was going on under the desk.

Now I've extended the fantasy to the idea of actually being seen, maybe from a distance, maybe through a window, maybe in the back row of a cinema. Since I've been in a relationship we actually include this in our lovemaking. Sometimes we actually play out little role plays. For instance, I've gone to a doctor, and he becomes the doctor and has to examine me. But very often we don't actually play it out, it's just that we talk it through while we're making love. We'll pretend we're on the back row of a cinema and we're having sex, and perhaps I'm masturbating him and he is me, and we start to say 'look, the usherette's seen us' and then we pretend we don't care and we just carry on, and we realise somebody else in the row has seen us. All this just heightens the feelings for us.

I'm sure there must be a deep psychological reason for all this. It may be something that appeals to the child in us – that as children we're told 'don't do that, don't play with yourself!' Sex was just not talked about at all at home. We were Anglo-Catholics. My mother was from a very Victorian family, very elderly parents with very Victorian values, and they were predominantly of a religious background. Many of her relatives were of the Church and it was all just very suppressed. So I think this idea of doing it with an audience is like the rebellious child who says, 'I know I'm not supposed to do this, so I'm going to do it, and everyone's going to see.' It's perhaps that I'm exerting my power over the situation. I'm a sexual being, and I'm going to do it whenever and wherever I want. There's certainly an element of that.

I often fantasise when I'm alone. I have masturbated in such a way that I can actually believe that I'm being touched by someone else. For example, I sometimes put a vibrator down my knickers and I pretend it's not there. I pretend I haven't put it there, and I'm getting the sensation from an outside force. And again, I sometimes hold conversations while I'm masturbating, pretty well along the lines of the interview situation. Or it could be going to confession, or something like that – anywhere there's a contradiction of formality on the surface, but in fact things aren't all they seem below decks. For me this just heightens it.

I have actually gone to the extent of virtually masturbating in public. When I was living in a basement flat a number of years ago, I was going through a particularly rampant stage and I was working in the theatre, so in the daytime I had a lot of time to myself. First of all I just started masturbating in all sorts of odd places, like in a closed wardrobe in the pitch dark, or under a table or in some very confined space. And then I just wanted to do it in more and more bizarre places. I got more and more courageous, and one day I got on the windowsill of the basement flat and did it in the window, with the intention that somebody hopefully would go by and just when they'd seen me for a split second, I'd duck so they wouldn't be quite sure whether they'd seen me or not. One day I was doing it and a number seven, or it might have been a number of nine, bus went by. I was living in a sort of apex of a triangle of houses and I think it was one of these empty buses – it might have been the end of the day – but the driver went round again to see if he could see me a second time! I don't think he was quite sure whether he'd seen it or not the first time, as I'd ducked down quite quickly, so he had to go round again. I wasn't doing it the second time.

I find that humour in sex, whether you're doing it on your own, or with another person, is vitally important. I think that's why I've been able to indulge these little fantasies for a long time. I've never felt guilty about them, I've just always felt the humour in the situation. Sometimes I quite like to make myself laugh when I'm having a wank, or when I'm just fantasising. Sometimes

64

the fantasies seem quite off the wall and I imagine that perhaps nobody else has these thoughts, but then it just makes me laugh.

I like the idea of wearing something quite formal, like a suit or a long skirt, and having this invisible hand going up my skirt. And I'm just conducting my business as normal, as though it's not happening. I can feel it, but I'm not going to let on to the rest of the world that I can. That's quite an interesting fantasy really. It's the idea that we are all able to assume various personas – we can be professional people, we can be barristers standing up in court – but underneath all that we're all sexual beings as well.

And sometimes I'm just tempted by the notion of bringing the two things together. I think it's quite common. I understand that in sex shops and through mail order catalogues and things you can buy special beads which you insert in your vagina, so that you get excited as you walk around, and somebody's got to be buying these things. Personally I don't actually like that idea, because I think there's something quite unclean about it. Like a lot of women, I suffer from thrush quite a bit, and I'm sure it would give me an attack of thrush. Some people wear special rubber underwear with protuberances that rub them as they walk around, and I suppose that's quite exciting. But I've always preferred, with the exception of the vibrator, to create my own environments, without resorting to stuff that you buy over a counter.

I do actually like tying myself up when I masturbate, and I imagine that somebody else has tied me up. I sometimes tie myself in knots, and I tie my hands together to make it very difficult for myself, and again it's the feeling that somebody else has done it to me which excites me. I have discovered fairly recently, now that I'm in a relationship with somebody that I really trust, that I actually enjoy being tied up by him. But I've been sexually active for about twenty years, and it's taken till now to find somebody I trust enough. But it's terribly exciting, and it's also quite liberating in a funny kind of way, because although you're tied up, you can be the sole recipient of the pleasure. And because you're tied up, there's no responsibility on you to pleasure your partner, so you can just lie back and enjoy it without any distractions. That's quite liberating, and I do find it very thrilling. I don't have to be terribly responsive, either with my body or with my hands. I don't have to attempt to pleasure him.

I think a lot of women find receiving quite difficult. Because we're generally the nurturers in a relationship, we tend to want to give, and I think women enjoy giving and feeling guilty if they're not giving. There have been times when I've been receiving a lot of pleasure, but I've had to break my concentration because I've got to return the pleasure by stimulating my partner; whereas when you're tied up you don't have to at all, you can't, so it intensifies the pleasure and it's liberating. My particular partner and I imagine quite a number of men find it exciting. But in fact when I do this with my partner I'm not tied that tightly, so there is a get-out if I wanted it. I wouldn't like to be manacled; it's more the suggestion in my mind, the fantasy of helplessness. I'm not into extreme things like being throttled to death, and I'm not into pain either. I just think it should be fun, it should be playful, and it should be risqué.

I'm sure we all have fantasies. Some of us want to play out the fantasies, and some of us never get to play them out. In my case, I had a kind of set of fantasies programmed into me, and because I've played nearly all of them out now – always the same ones, the exhibitionist one, and the risk of being caught thing – I don't feel I need to do them so much any more. The other thing I have actually done, which links up to the fantasy of being behind a desk, is that in a working situation, in an office where people were walking in and out, and walking past the door, I have actually masturbated. I find it so exciting to think that there's only a desk that separates me from being caught, and even then I might still be caught because somebody might come right over and find out what I'm doing, or they might come into the office too quickly. I might have lost my job, but it was worth it, it was such a turn-on.

I love the idea of rocking the boat, and so I have on a couple of occasions when I've actually been in a place of employment where the atmosphere is a little bit formal and there are certain roles that you have to play. When the boss, or everybody else, has gone out for an hour, I just lie on the floor in the boss's office and have a wank. And again, there's a fairly low risk of being caught, because you know they've gone out, but it's more sort of, 'You think this office is so formal, if you only knew what was going on when your back was turned.' It's that kind of thing, just shaking the social mores a bit. But there have been one or two situations like that.

These are my main fantasies: this idea of the risk of being caught, and actually being caught. In my childhood I was nearly caught a couple of times by my father, because he always used to walk around on silent feet – it was almost as if he was on oiled wheels. A couple of times he would walk into a room and I'd have to suddenly pull on my clothes, but I think I had that fantasy before I remember being caught. I do remember being seen by somebody I was staying with when I was on holiday in France one year. They walked past an open window, looked in, and I was masturbating. But again I think the idea was there before that.

I actually didn't become sexually aware until surprisingly late for somebody who likes sex a great deal, as I do. I didn't become aware that I had a clitoris until I was nearly seventeen, and it was because a man happened to touch me there, otherwise I don't know when I would have found it. Somebody masturbated me to orgasm in a car once, and that was what started me off masturbating. I just thought it was fantastic – I don't know what it was, I don't understand it, but I'm going to do it again – that was when it all started really.

I've been lucky enough to be with a man who will fantasise with me. To begin with I led the fantasies and he responded, but I think it's obviously something he had a latent desire to do, because now he's started to initiate them and I respond to him. So our fantasies fuel each other's. And I've introduced him to things I've discovered only quite recently, things like crotchless panties. It always seems a bit of a joke – crotchless panties are the sort of thing Joan Collins gets at Christmas – but I actually decided to buy a pair, about a year ago, and they were so exciting. I nearly went through the roof with excitement the first time we used them. And he enjoyed that, and suggested, 'Why don't you go and buy a rubber suit from Ann Summers, or perhaps we could go and choose one together?', so he's quite into all of that. His fantasies are actually an extension of my own fantasies, which is lovely. I'm lucky enough to have met somebody whose fantasies coincide with mine. He likes the risk of being caught fantasy, and shocking people, and the usherette at the cinema. I just think that the relationship is so good on so many levels that the sex is not excluded from that.

THE MIDDLE-CLASS
APPEAL

The Middle-Class Appeal

The English middle class has a reputation for being a bastion of the well ordered and the mundane. But beneath the surface veneer lie the surprises.

Jane is one of the few women whose fantasies are included in this book who comes from a liberal background. Her parents encouraged her to experiment with sex and romance as a teenager, and her sexual fantasies reflect a balance of understanding and experience.

Alice also feels at one and content with her sexuality. She came out as a lesbian when she was twenty-three and was able to tell her parents about it. Her fantasies involve the risqué element of being seen making love in public places. Enjoying the sensation of being watched, she craves attention.

Susan, on the other hand, comes from a family where there was no talk about sex at all, and she was left to her own devices to discover the necessary information. Her sexual fantasies only developed when she had learned to cope with her parentally imposed Catholic guilt. Early fantasies were predominantly romantic. Now single and in her mid-thirties, she has sexual fantasies in which she relives sexual encounters with past and present boyfriends.

Pamela married young and was divorced two years later. She came from a family where sex was frowned upon, never discussed. She was brought up in a strict environment to be a 'nice, clean-living' girl, but she explains that what she finds sexually exciting are sleazy, unsavoury sexual scenarios – meeting 'dirty old men' in parks, for instance. Her more extreme fantasies now involve the idea of sexual contact with dogs.

Alex likes the anonymity of city life, so that she can experiment sexually without exciting comment. Her fantasies revolve around sado-masochistic scenarios. Her desire is to explore the outer limits of her threshold for pain.

Jane aged 31

I come from a very liberal home, so sex was never frightening and never not allowed. In retrospect, I could have done with a bit more rule telling, because my parents used to let me bring boyfriends home. I had a boyfriend when I was seventeen who my parents would let me bring home, and we'd sleep together and he'd stay the night. In comparison to my peers and my best friend, I actually started relatively late with all that, but people I've met since have said, 'Oh, you were starting with boys and doing rude things very young.' At that stage I didn't make much time for fantasy as I was doing all sorts of capers, even at fourteen, fifteen. I was never told it was naughty or wrong.

By the time I was fifteen I was going to parties and getting off with people and going into bedrooms with them, and going to bed with them really and doing everything but have full penetrative sex. I think I was just quite sexual as a kid. I never told my parents I was doing all that sort of stuff, but as soon as I started going out with someone, they knew. I always thought sex was quite good fun. I never thought that it was wrong or felt guilty about it. I feel much more guilty about it now when I do it, because I know more about what's involved now. My dad always used to refer to us as being like puppies. He used to say, 'You have to do those things when you're growing up, because you're just like puppies, you're finding out.'

I suppose there was an element that was vaguely sordid, because I was having it off with all sorts of people. Occasionally it would be the same person twice. Between the ages of fifteen and seventeen there were quite a lot of boys I gave blow jobs to and let them put their hand down my knickers and all sorts of stuff like that, and I didn't really go out with them. Some of them were really good friends of mine, so that was nice, but some were just people I met, including total strangers, which was fairly horrendous. Even then I knew that that was unpleasant and unrewarding. When I was with boys that I knew who were quite sexy I enjoyed it. I used to get drunk a lot at that time as well, which I thought was quite racy. Considering I came from nice middle-class background, I behaved in a downmarket way – like an 'Essex girl'. Perhaps that's what I am, a 'middle-class Essex girl'.

By the time I was seventeen I considered that I knew what I was doing, and I'd had enough of the playing around. I'd had full sex once at this point, with a complete stranger. Then I started going out with a boy who's still a friend today, and we were together for a couple of years. That relationship was all very nice and sweet and jolly and comforting, good jolly sex.

I don't remember having sexual fantasies early on. I always was quite a sexual person, in that I started doing things from a young age. I think I felt that my sexual imagination was concentrated on things that I already knew and was just an extension of that. I had a very straightforward idea of sex. I thought it was all fine and good, nothing horrible. My brother had a big stack of pornographic magazines, and I remember looking at them and thinking they had no connection with reality at all. I didn't really find the pictures at all interesting. They turned me on, but after a while I went off them, thinking they were sordid and horrible. My sexual fantasies just became related to things I already knew from doing really basic, simple things with boys, though in the fantasies there were more of these things. I liked to have more sex and do more things than the people I was with, so it was all extended in my head.

I always fantasised about people I knew, sometimes people I fancied but couldn't go out with. I imagined what it would be like and what I'd do and things like that. I can remember when I was about thirteen that I'd never had anybody touch my breasts, and then finally somebody did when I was about fourteen and he took my top off and licked my bosoms, and I can remember thinking that this was how I'd imagined it; this was deeply exciting and wonderful and I wanted to do some more of it. That was all we did on that occasion, but I can remember imagining what it would be like if he'd done more of that and in different places, and how nice that was.

I don't have sex very often these days. I don't have a partner, and I haven't had a partner for years. Sometimes I have vague liaisons, smashing into someone in the middle of the night. Most of my sexual fantasies involve people I know or have known. I lie in bed before I go to sleep, or sometimes I lie in bed in the mornings fantasising about past sex. I give myself a treat time of imagining very nice sex. I'd imagine a scenario, and who I was with, then I'd imagine where we were. I quite like the idea of sex in public, or having someone grope me in the cinema or the back of a taxi, things like that. He would make me come with his hand while we were in public places. It is always someone I know and usually quite nice.

I used to really like the boring domestic detail of it. I loved to fantasise about sitting up in the kitchen, having sex on a kitchen chair. My fantasies involve quite a lot of conversation as well – what you'd say to someone, and how you get round to it. You'd arrive home, and you'd go into the kitchen, and you'd start hugging and kissing and then you'd sit down on top of each other and start licking each other, and tearing some clothes off, but not bothering to take all your clothes off, so you'd have half your clothes on. I imagine it all happening very slowly, and take my time over the fantasy. That is the joy of doing it, not just having a wank – you could spend hours thinking about it and planning it and then have the wank.

My fantasies are to do with the normal things that people like, at least what I think is normal. My kitchen fantasy involves a completely normal domestic situation. I used to quite like to imagine having a lot of sex all through the day. So you'd be doing things like having your breakfast, or reading the Sunday papers, and you'd start rubbing the man's inner thigh with your leg while you're sitting there, and then you'd start fiddling about with your foot on his prick. Then you'd start doing other things – you'd sit astride him, and then you'd be sitting on the chair and he'd kneel down in front of you and be sucking and licking you. I always want a lot of sex, and I worry that men think that it's a bit overwhelming, so I imagine I'm with someone who wants to have a hell of a lot of sex, so that whenever you say, 'Lets do it in the kitchen and let's do it on the stairs, and let's do it wherever . . .' it's not a problem.

I go through the order of what I'd like done to me in bed. I imagine that somebody is there, and we undress each other and we start doing a lot of sloppy, slobbery kissing, and then I give a blow job. I always love giving a lot of blow jobs. I quite like blokes' bums, so I like the idea of licking their bums and to have them lick me.

I like to remember nice sex that I've had, and to relive it in my mind. For me that's often centred around food – going to bed with lots of food like strawberries and chocolate and cake, feeding each other while you're fucking. I think that there's something sensuous about lovely food, so I use those experiences from my sex life to get off when I'm on my own. I never fantasise about coming. I fantasise about all the things leading up to it, not penetration, but all the other things you can do, like licking men's thighs. All my fantasies are quite cosy and comfy really!

I find fantasising quite a good way of relaxing. I like to fantasise sometimes that I'm half awake and an ex-boyfriend appears in my bed and is fucking me slowly and gently. It can be very comforting. But I suppose you could get to the stage where you're thinking about it too much, especially if you haven't had sex for a long time, and sometimes it makes me worse, more horny, and I've got nowhere I can go with it apart from myself. And sometimes I think that's pointless and I stop myself.

Alice aged 27

It became clear to me quite early on that I was into women. Somewhere between the ages of eleven and thirteen, I began to suspect that there was something different about me. I grew up in a small town where there was nobody like me to identify with, so I tried to keep my feelings secret for quite a long time. I came out as a lesbian, and told a close friend, when I was sixteen. But I was twenty-three when I told my parents, and it was very, very important to me to make this statement to them, and to go ahead and live my own life.

I never had any problems being a lesbian. The problem for me was in finding a community where I could fit in. I felt quite isolated for many years, but at the time I just thought that this was the price you've got to pay, and I was more than willing to. I have never tried to convince myself that I'm not a lesbian. I was always quite happy with the way I felt and I just tried to deal with the problems as they arose. Now I live in a small town in a comparatively strong community, and I make the most of my gay and lesbian friends here, and I hope to stay here. It makes me feel stronger as an individual to be in a close community.

I have been through different phases in my sexual life and my sexual fantasies have changed over the years, and they're constantly changing. I can't just say that there are a couple of fantasies that recur over and over again; they're actually all over the place. They're to do with what I do on a daily basis. If I go clubbing, and I find a woman incredibly attractive and beautiful, then I'll come home and think about it.

Years ago, when I was not really out and I didn't know any lesbians, the women in my fantasies didn't have any faces, they were just blank. But for the last four or five years, since I've been enjoying an active sex life, there are particular women I find attractive, and they are all gay women who appear in my fantasies. I've never even thought about straight women, because I'm not out there trying to convince as many straight women as possible of how much fun lesbian sex could be. I just cling to the community and the people and the style and the codes. This is very important to me, and it's actually what I'm attracted to.

My sexual fantasies happen as a kind of daydream, rather

than that I go to bed and turn myself on. They happen every-where. Sometimes I'll just sit at my desk and start fantasising. There are various stories that I think about, and they are con-stantly changing and developing. The simplest one is that I imagine going out, meeting a woman and finding the courage to engage her in conversation. I dance with her and we are getting closer and closer. It's not so much that I want to fuck her silly – there's a lot of emotion, and I take my time kissing and touching whilst we are actually in the club. I find it a turn-on that we are being watched by other women there, not in a straight place, but in the security of a gay club or bar, where I know there's not going to be any disturbance.

On the other hand, my fantasies also go to the other extreme, where I go to public places, and I think of going down on a woman in front of straight people. It could be anywhere – it could be in a phone box, or on a train, or it could be in a public toilet.

I fantasise about men as well, and I want to say here that I was quite confused about this at the beginning, but there are books about it. From reading these books I discovered that quite a few women who identify themselves as lesbians do have these fantasies. This made me feel more secure and less guilty, though I didn't exactly feel guilty, as after all my fantasies are my fanta-sies and I don't share them with anyone; but I was surprised. I thought, how strange. To start with I wondered if I might be in-terested in men, but I knew I was not. But I thought there was still no reason not to have the fantasy.

It's kind of a turn-on to imagine that I'm having sex with a woman, and that a man, or men, are watching. There are no faces and they don't get close to us, and they don't really inter-fere or take part in this. I don't want to shock them, but I find it very exciting. They are not particularly gay or straight men, just men who get aroused by watching me fucking another woman, and this in turn turns me on. But the men hardly ever interfere – they want to, and I know they want to, but I won't allow it. This is somehow attention-seeking on my part, and a kind of teasing. I enjoy saying no. But I don't get a kick out of the idea of fucking a man. I don't find it at all arousing. The man might want to touch and feel and join in, but in my mind I don't give him the possibi-lity.

My other fantasies involve a bit of what some people might call S & M. I imagine tying women up, using restraints, or the other way round, being tied up. It's always about only one other woman. She would be restraining me, and teasing me. The point is that I'm helpless. It's a kind of trust thing – I like the feeling that I can trust this woman, that I'm putting myself into her hands, letting her do the playing without me being able to interfere. I feel a lot of tension – what is she going to do next? It could be oral sex, or some sort of penetration. I'm not into vegetables, but I like fisting.

I don't stop fantasising after I've reached a mental climax. It goes on, I think about it endlessly. We're lying together on the bed, or on a chair, or better still, a kitchen table – I love the idea of fucking another woman on the kitchen table, slowly, in all sorts of positions. This doesn't actually make me come. A minute later I might go back to my computer and type an essay. It gives me a relaxing break to fantasise like this when I'm working hard and stressed out. I'll sit back and have a cigarette, listen to music on the radio and relax into my fantasy.

My masturbatory fantasies are more immediately sexual, more straightforward. It depends on my mood. Sometimes I like to masturbate and just lie there for an hour, a couple of hours just thinking about sex, and trying to visualise a particular woman's face, and her body, and slowly, slowly getting more aroused. I'm using some sort of toy, a vibrator, or a dildo, anything I can find. I learned how to masturbate after I came out. I didn't do it beforehand. I never even thought of it, which I find quite strange now. I only started after talking to a lot of women about it, and then I realised what a wonderful thing it is – you can do it whenever and wherever you want to! At the beginning I felt a bit odd about doing it, sometimes five times a day, and sometimes only once in two weeks. I've gradually accepted it as just a fun thing to do, and it's about taking care of myself, exploring myself, liking myself, which is very important. It's still a learning process for me. There are still new things to discover. Talking about it with friends helps a lot. And I'm much more aware of my body since I started doing it.

There's a difference between masturbating and having sex with another woman. With another woman you can neglect your

79

own body to a greater or lesser extent, but if you're masturbating you have to come to terms with your body. I'm getting more and more into masturbation. Sometimes I feel I'd rather do it myself because I know exactly what I want now, here, how far I want to go. Then the fantasies just come. Sometimes I find it arousing to think about fucking a man. I'm very much in control, and I get off on it. I couldn't imagine doing it in real life, there's a big difference, and I've come to terms with it.

There's a lot of pressure and prejudice about women fucking other women, with dildoes or strap-ons or whatever it is, but what I do in real life and in my fantasies isn't really about the penis; it's just a toy, and people should just face it, and accept the way I am. It's not a substitute, it's something I choose, and there are many things you can do with it. People say that any kind of penetration is simulating heterosexual sex – obviously they don't know what they're talking about. I've never slept with men, but I've come very, very close to it. At certain stages of my life I've thought that I might be attracted to men, and partly I've wanted this. It would have made my life easier. But very quickly I realised that no, there is no need to force myself to prove that I'm a lesbian, that I don't want to sleep with men.

Susan aged 35

I had a very restrictive upbringing. Both my parents were quite old – thirty-eight – when they had me. They're from a completely different generation. My mother was brought up in the Midlands in a Victorian family with very strong principles, so she was particularly inhibited. My father was also a very shy man. The way I was taught about sex was that my mother thrust a book into my hands and said, 'Here, read this. If you've got any questions ask me.' And disappeared. That was my sex education, and I was too shy to ask any questions. That was when I was fourteen, and it took me years of talking to my sisters and listening to any gossip I could pick up at school – which was all wrong, babies coming out of your belly button and so on – to find out. Sexual intercourse really wasn't discussed until I was working. I started working when I was fifteen and I learnt what was going on through going to night clubs and the conversations we had as girls in the ladies' room. Also there were young women falling pregnant around me which gave me some idea.

My early sexual dreams were quite frightening, because I'd had that very strict Catholic upbringing where men only want to get to know you because they're going to rape you. They're going to stick their thing in you and get you pregnant, and that's all they want from you. So I was quite nervous about sex. I thought that sex was going to be violent, a violent encounter. My parents never showed any outward signs of affection in front of us children. There was no hugging and kissing or any of that, though there might have been a quick peck on the cheek. So we were not shown any kind of example, which left me totally confused. I think I blocked out the idea of fantasies at that early stage.

I started fantasising in a very romantic way when, as a teenager, I began going out in a gang of girls. My fantasy was that a young man was going to come along and it was going to be love and courting and eventually they'd ask you to marry them and you'd have the big traditional wedding, which most of my young friends went through, and set up house together and live happily ever after. Very Mills and Boon. Most of my contemporaries are now divorced; very few of them are still married. They lived that

81

dream and have moved on to the next husband, even the fourth one by now, and have children by each husband.

My real sexual fantasies only started much later. I was twenty when I lost my virginity, and it was a real snatch and grab affair. It wasn't at all romantic, so my illusion was ruined. I hadn't had any sex education, so I didn't know about condoms or what I could use. I had no protection, so it was all very risky. I lived like that for quite some time, still very nervous about dealing with men. Then I met someone who was a little bit more stable and we started to live together, and that's when I began to learn a lot more through him. I was very naive.

When I was about twenty-two I had a relationship with a man ten years older than me, and that changed my attitudes. He was far more experienced than I was, a real womaniser, so he knew how to please a woman, though it was still really a learning process for me. I did have some fantasies with him but it was still a very dangerous relationship with him, because he was able to manipulate me, through very exciting physical pleasure. I didn't realise until years later that I was being manipulated – that I was putting my trust in him, but to him I was just a toy. That was quite painful, because I'd been brought up with this romantic notion that you would develop a relationship with the man and that you would settle down and get married, and have children. None of that was forthcoming, so my romantic fantasies were shattered.

After that I had a seven-year relationship with a really boring man. It would have taken a rugby team to get me going with this chap, he was just very boring!

I'm a late developer. Recently I think I've come to terms with my sexuality. I've started to understand my sexuality as a woman, and to know what pleasure I want from a man. And I've found men who have as strong a character as I have. Most men I scare and inhibit, because my fantasies and my desires can really unnerve them. If I throw them on the bed, or off the bed, if I come over too physical, they can be quite taken aback.

I'm quite big myself, and I fantasise about big men. They have to be strong, probably because for seven years I put up with a weak man, and I know that I totally screwed him up. After him, I knew that I'd need someone who was both physically and mentally strong. I met two men at that time who both wanted to get involved with me, and I just went along for the ride. They were both very big men, over six foot. In a way they were just as screwed up as everybody else, but physically big and quite sure of themselves. The confidence was important to me. Now I fantasise about men. They can be from any walk of life, but they have to be big and confident, and they take control of me physically and mentally. Normally I fantasise about making love with the people I'm involved with or those I used to be involved with.

There is one particular ex-boyfriend from years ago who went to Australia, I often fantasise about him. In fact I often call his name out loud when I'm actually making love with someone else – a big mistake, it ruins their rhythm. This happened to me recently on a one-night stand, when I went off into a fantasy about the previous lover. I was not long out of the seven-year relationship and felt like a virgin with this different man. He said to me, 'you need sorting out, come over and I'll sort you out', and I went, but my mind was miles away. At one point he held me at arm's length and said, 'you're thinking about someone else', and I said, 'What do you expect? You're a total stranger.' He was a black man, born in England, but his parents were from Jamaica, and since that night I've had quite a lot of fantasies about black men. I'm attracted to their character. They're very strong men, very direct, and there's no pretence. If they want sex they'll just phone me up at work and say, what are you doing tonight? Can I come round? And I'll just say yes or no. If it suits me they come round.

I think I've been fantasising about that openness, and that directness, and about the way that we met. One of the two black guys I met recently was a cameraman, and I had to sort out his passport for a trip abroad. When I got the passport I saw his photograph, where he looked very handsome. Also I had his height and his age – we were a very similar age, and he was about six foot four. So I had the basic images to fantasise about. Then the telephone conversations started, which were very sexual, very suggestive. And those phone calls increased the fantasy about this man. I had a voice and a name, and this picture. It all came together in my mind.

One day he just turned up in my office out of the blue, and he seemed to have been having the same fantasy as I'd been having. So we decided we wanted to live this fantasy. But he went off filming. When he came back, I met him at the airport, and then I was very distant and disappeared. Then I got a phone call out of the blue inviting me round. He seemed to have had quite a fantasy about me. He'd thought about me when he was away, and there were things that he'd remembered about me. My fantasy was that it would be a very physical relationship, and that's what happened. It was very exclusive, and lived up to everything we'd both fantasised about. Though the relationship didn't really continue, I fantasise about it in minute detail quite often.

The other black guy was Cuban originally, and again was very direct. My fantasies always have a lot to do with their personalities and are always about people I'm involved with. In my fantasies I actually live the life of being with this person. It's not just the sexual part, it's the whole package, day-to-day scenarios, such as going to the cinema, what we've done that night or that weekend. Or if we've had sex in reality then I relive that. Because these are not easy relationships – they're both involved with someone else – I also fantasise about their relationships with the other women. By chance I happen to know who they are and have met them, and I find myself fantasising about their day-to-day lives with the men in my life.

Most of these fantasies are thought about in the middle of the night, when I'm half asleep. I don't sit and fantasise during the day time, so often they're not very clear to me, other than the re-living. Sometimes I imagine where I might meet up with lovers, in the backs of cars or in parks or in surreal situations in public – not really to put on a public display, but to do it out in the open. Once on holiday in Australia with a boyfriend we were out in a speedboat with no one for miles, so we took all our clothes off and made love in the boat all afternoon. Suddenly we realised that all these other boats had gradually drifted in, because all they could see were our bums going up and down. They knew exactly what was happening, and we'd been giving a performance all afternoon. We were so engrossed that we didn't realise what was going on until we eventually put our heads up. They were virtually holding signs up giving points. Very embarrassing! I still fantasise about that incident. I think I enjoyed the encounter.

That boyfriend was the one who set the ground rules for my sexual pleasure. I think most women go through life not knowing how to have an orgasm. I learnt late, though still at a fairly young age, what pleasure your body can give you. He showed me that, and that's a problem I've had with other men: I know what it could be like and they don't know what to do, they're fumbling. It's a big problem for a lot of men. I suppose my fantasies are often based on my experiences with him, and knowing what pleasure I had with that confident man.

The way I got through seven years of a bad relationship was to superimpose the face of the man who did know how to turn me on and imagine the sex was with him. The problem I've always had with fantasy is that, because I had strict Catholic upbringing, fantasies always seemed to me to be wrong, and when I have them I feel guilty. Over the last couple of years I have begun to feel less guilty and fantasise more. It was always classed as dirty when I was growing up. The Catholic notion was that you would be punished, and were committing a sin. I'd have to go and tell the priest that I had this dream, so it's been very difficult. But now I've been able to throw all that indoctrination out and am able to deal with my own sexuality.

Pamela aged 38

We were a family who didn't talk about sex. I remember when I was about seven or eight going to see a James Bond film, and obviously the word sexy was used in this James Bond film. I came home and told my parents, isn't Sean Connery sexy, and was given such a telling off for using the word sexy and told never to use the word again. Sex wasn't discussed. I never saw my parents without their clothes on. They were quite liberal in other ways, but sex was something which greatly embarrassed them, and they didn't tell me anything about it, even about my periods. I was quite lucky in that I had older friends, I knew quite a lot, and I went to a school where we were actually taught sex education, so I never felt that there was anything I didn't know, but it didn't come from my parents. It was fairly religious on my mother's side, so I didn't believe in sex before marriage when I was very young. I certainly thought I would wait until I got married to have sex.

When I was about thirteen, and some of the girls in my class were starting to experiment with sex, I remember thinking it was wrong, that they shouldn't do that. I was a bit prim and proper about sex at that stage, although I was interested in boys from about twelve or thirteen. And I had boyfriends from thirteen. I was quite grown up looking, I looked a lot older than my age. I had long blonde hair and black eye make-up and could pass for somebody a lot older, so I went into discos and pubs from about that age. My boyfriends were around my age, and were probably as inexperienced, so there was no great pressure.

I had my first really steady boyfriend at fifteen. He later became my husband, though we divorced after two years. He was my first sexual partner before marriage. I was only fifteen when I lost my virginity, and it was the most horrendous experience of my life. We'd been going out together for about a year, and doing some petting, and the petting was building up. I was intrigued and interested in sex, but a bit frightened of going the full way. After all, I had this vision that I would marry and be a virgin on my wedding night.

One day we'd been out to a disco, and we'd been drinking. He was a virgin as well, and three years older than me. We'd both been drinking heavily and had a Chinese meal, never the order to do things in – dancing, drinking, meal. We came home and the petting went a bit further, and I said to him, yeah, OK, let's go the full way. This was on the floor, in front of the fire, on a sheepskin rug in my parent's living room while they were in bed. He was so excited at the prospect of this. It was his first time as well, and we'd been building up over a year. It wasn't painful – it was over and done with in two seconds, just two strokes. I bled profusely, and the sight of the blood, the excitement and the shock of it all made him throw up all over me. After that I wasn't keen at all. I thought, well, if that's it, I can do without it. So we didn't actually do it again for quite some months, and it was never good. This was probably one of the main reasons for the marriage break-up.

I masturbated from as early as I can remember – I can't remember not doing it, even when I was a baby. I remember once being caught by my mother, and being smacked and told this was terrible and I must never do it again. But I continued to do it, without admitting it to anybody. I remember always having sexual feelings, I can't remember a time when I didn't. I had an older brother who was eight years older than me, and I remember finding some dirty magazines like *Playboy* that he had in his early teens, and I used to be fascinated. When everyone was out I'd go and look at these dirty magazines, possibly because we didn't talk about sex, but I was also very intrigued. I always wanted to know, and any opportunity of finding out anything about it, from a programme or movie, was very welcome. I could get into X-rated movies from about the age of twelve, so I used to go and see *Up The Junction* and all those types of films in the late sixties, because I was terribly intrigued about sex and always felt sexual. I was a tomboy when I was growing up, and I liked to play with boys in a competitive way. I wasn't very feminine. By the time I was twelve my interest had changed and I definitely viewed boys in a sexual way. I've had quite strong sexual urges for as long as I can remember.

My earliest fantasies were always about men – I wasn't ever interested in girls or women – and they were purely about the sex act, before I knew how awful it was! The fantasies were about penetration, and also the curiosity about a man's body, because I hadn't actually seen a man's body. I hadn't seen my father or my brother or anybody else. And rather than me doing something in my fantasies, I always waned things done to me. I wanted people to touch me, probably covertly, with me standing there not having anything to do with it, just having somebody pamper me. This is still part of the fantasy I have now, but it has probably always been there. Then penetration became important. Although I wanted to wait, it intrigued me.

My fantasies have changed a bit over the years, though some of them have followed through. When I was quite young I remember seeing an Emmanuelle film, around thirteen or fourteen. The girl in the film was in Japan and she went with her boyfriend to a massage parlour. It was very old-fashioned with marble walls and marble slabs, and the two of them were massaged by two very beautiful Japanese women. They were brought to orgasm and then they ended up having sex together afterwards. That became a fantasy for me for a long time, being massaged by a Japanese woman, and it can only have been because of the film, because I found it very erotic. I fantasised about a similar scenario.

Strangely enough, later in life, when I was in my twenties, I was staying with a girlfriend in Switzerland, and she said to me, 'What would you like to do? Is there something we can arrange that you'd really like to do?' So I said, just as a joke, that I'd really like to have an erotic massage. She said that she knew someone in a hotel who could do that. It was a five star hotel with a health club, and she arranged a massage. To this day I don't know whether it just happened or whether it was something that she actually arranged, but I went to have the massage, given by an ugly, short, little Italian man, and he gave me the most wonderful massage I've ever had in my life, without actually stimulating me anywhere in particular. It was such an erotic massage that he brought me to orgasm twice. I felt I'd lived out a fantasy. Although it wasn't exactly the fantasy I'd had all those years, I felt I had partially lived it out.

There are other fantasies I have which I would actually be repulsed by in reality, and wouldn't want to carry out. During the sex act, if I think about these fantasies they turn me on more than anything else, but they are things I wouldn't do. There are several. One is really quite revolting. It's been around for a lot of years, and I don't really know where it comes from. I'm walking through a park, quite a public place, in the daylight, and there's an old man, a dirty old man with a mac on. He's quite old, and he asks me to sit down beside him. I sit down and he starts to touch me up. I just sit there and I let him. He doesn't have sex with me, he just touches me up. He uses various things to touch me up with – it might be his walking stick, or some other thing he has on him. I don't actually climax in my fantasy, and he doesn't actually have full sex with me. I visualise him as being quite dirty and smelly. Sometimes I fantasise the same thing in a men's toilet. The dirtier, the grubbier the situation, the more erotic I find it. If I'm having sex and I think of this fantasy, it turns me on.

The only things I can think of that might explain this fantasy is that I can remember being about seven and being in a park with a friend, and old man with a dog came along. We were talking to his dog and he was getting us to bend over the seat. I don't think I was aware of what was going on, and I can't remember him touching either of us. In retrospect, I think he was just trying to look at our knickers. I think my fantasy has just grown from the idea and the memory of this, looking back, although because I wasn't really sexually aware at the time, it is hard for me to believe that my fantasies come from that – I wasn't turned on by the situation at the time.

On a couple of occasions when I was young, men flashed at me from outside public toilets and in public parks as well, and I remember once going back to see if I could catch a glimpse, see what it looked like.

I used to have a fantasy about a threesome, always me with an older man and an older woman, probably a married couple, and they'd pick me up and take me somewhere and seduce me. I would be very much on the receiving end. I'm lying back quietly and they're doing all sorts of things to me. I once followed this up and did have a threesome with a man and a woman, but I found that I wasn't turned on by this at all really. I wasn't interested in touching the other woman, and I wasn't particularly interested in her touching me. I think I felt a bit jealous as well. So that's a fantasy that doesn't turn me on very much any more, because I pursued it and it didn't give me the same exciting feeling I had imagined.

I often fantasise about being taken, and not having much part in it, but never about being raped. I like to fantasise about groups of people taking me, and even tying me up, men or women, they're just touching me all over and giving me pleasure, teasing me. Although they're taking me, it's not rape. I couldn't think about that. I also fantasise about big black men, assuming that it's all true – that black men are much more well-endowed than white men. Usually in the fantasies there are two or three of these big men. It has to be a lot to make it exciting, different to real life.

I once had an experience with two men that I was travelling with. We were travelling overland, and they climbed into my sleeping bag one night and started to tease me, one starting at my head and one starting at my toes and meeting in the middle. It was very erotic, and I got turned on a lot, and then I suddenly got a bit frightened. After all, I had to see them the next day. I thought, I don't know how far I want this to go. What will it be like to face them in the morning if it goes too far? We were sleeping on the beach, so I said, let's all go for a swim and cool off, and we'll think about this later. We all went for a swim, and they never came back. They went off and had a thing together – apparently they were bisexual. They didn't come back until next day. Since then I've had a fantasy about two men pampering me. I'm not sure that penetration comes into it. Sometimes it does, but that's not the important part of the fantasy. In all my fantasies I'm either lying there, or sitting there or standing there not doing anything, and somebody's just giving me complete enjoyment.

This is possibly because most of the men that I have had relationships with, with the exception of my current lover, who is completely different, have been quite selfish, not very good lovers, ultimately only interested in their own orgasm. I have faked so many orgasms, I can't remember the number of times I've done it. It's basically because I've got bored and wanted to get it over and done with. I've had so many experiences with men who aren't good lovers, even though I've tried to tell them what I would like to do and what I would like done, and I've always been the one who's done all the giving. So my fantasies have been the opposite, with me not doing anything or contributing

90

anything, just enjoying them. Though with my current lover, who is amazing and wouldn't dream of having an orgasm until I'm fully satisfied, I still have the fantasies when he's making love to me, I'm not quite sure why. Perhaps it's to heighten the feeling, but it's probably not necessary any more.

I don't think I fantasised when I was first seeing him, because he was such a breath of fresh air. Now we've been together for three years and I do. I'm sure he does too, but he doesn't admit to it. I know that like a lot of men he has a fantasy about a threesome, and he also fantasises about a row of naked women all bending over, and he goes along the line and has them one after the other. He tells me about it when we're making love.

I've recently started having fantasies about dogs. But not penetration. When I was a little girl we had a dog, a bitch, and we didn't have her doctored. She used to come on heat and all the dogs in the neighbourhood used to follow me to school. It used to be a nightmare, and my mother used to buy sprays and things to put over me. It was quite awful and I hated it, going to school with dogs following me like the Pied Piper. I remember once a dog doing its bit up my leg. I couldn't shake it off, but I was quite intrigued by its parts. Although I wished the dog would go away, as it was very embarrassing, I was intrigued by it.

Also, recently a friend told me a story. The story was that this girl was having a party thrown for her birthday, a surprise party in her house. She came in unexpectedly, and they were hiding in the lounge, her parents and her boyfriend and various friends that were throwing the surprise party. They heard her go into the kitchen, and they were waiting for her to come into the lounge because they were going to switch the lights on. But she didn't come in, so they waited a while. They could hear her in the kitchen and thought she was making a cup of coffee or something and were convinced she'd come into the lounge. She didn't come in, so after a while they thought, this is silly, we'll go and take the party out into the kitchen. They opened the kitchen door and she was lying on the floor smothered in dog food, with a dog licking the food off her. I remember thinking when I was told this story, this is so horrible. Everything about it was horrible: the embarrassment of everybody seeing you in this position, the very thought of having smelly dog food all over you, the thought of having a dog lick you on your most private parts. And yet there's something about it that intrigues me. Bestiality really does repulse me, but somehow the idea turns me on.

I think my dog has only recently come into my fantasies, and it's to do with the dirty old man in the mac – he's got a dog with him. I think it's sniffing more than anything else that does it for me. But I love the idea of animals. I read a story about a woman with a gorilla which I really loved, though it's horrible.

Fantasy is very different from reality. I try to think up the most gross things I can if I really want to heighten my sex life. Everything apart from pain, that is. Sado-masochism holds no attraction for me at all, not even in my fantasies. I can't associate that with something sexual. I can with dirt and grubbiness, and people who are dirty and grubby, and situations in toilets. I go into a ladies' toilet in a summer dress, and three very butch girls come in, and they're quite threatening and frightening. The leader tells the other two to hold the door to make sure that nobody comes in while she sexually abuses me. This quite appeals to me because I see it as being dirty. I like the thought of being tied up and having things done to me, maybe with several instruments, being in these situations and being with people I wouldn't normally have sex with.

When I was about nineteen, and in my first job, there was a chap who was in the art department of the company I worked for. He must have been about forty five, but at the time I thought that was very old. He was very unattractive – nice chap, but very unattractive. He was quite odd looking in a way, arty with messy hair, a bit like Worzel Gummidge, and I used to fantasise about having sex with him. There were two young men who worked in the department with him who I would have gone out with and fancied, but no, it was the unattractive one that I had sexual fantasies about. I do fantasise about people who I wouldn't ever be attracted to in real life. I used to blush when I saw him because I could picture the fantasies I'd had the night before, and I used to think that he'd know. Had he ever made a pass at me I would have run a mile, but I couldn't stop fantasising about him.

I come from a nice, clean middle-class background, and I think in a way I like the sordid idea of dirt as a response to that and to the fact that sex wasn't discussed, my naughty secret.

I lived out somebody's sexual fantasy once, which was a bizarre and potentially dangerous thing to do, because I thought it would be exciting and I thought it would become my fantasy. It started with a crossed line on the telephone at work. I got talking to this chap, and I don't remember how it developed, but he rang me back another time and it built up. I can't remember why, but we started to talk about sex. He said to me, I've got this sexual fantasy, and this is what it is. He told me his sexual fantasy was that a woman he'd never met before and didn't know would come into his flat. He'd have all the lights turned off, and a bottle of champagne by his bedside. She'd come into his flat, not turn the lights on, so he wouldn't see her face and she wouldn't see his, it would be complete darkness, and she'd take all her clothes off and get into bed with him. Then they would pet. They wouldn't have full sex, and they wouldn't speak a word. They'd drink a glass of champagne, then she would put her clothes on and she would leave, not one word having passed between them. And I said to him OK. It was about eight years ago, and I don't know why I agreed to do it. He told me his address, told me he would leave the latch on, told me which room he'd be in, where to find it.

When I went, it was in complete darkness. I couldn't see his face, didn't know him at all. We didn't actually have penetrative sex, but we did pet. I did do what he'd said, and we had the glass of champagne, and we uttered not one word. It was pitch darkness. If he walked into this room now I wouldn't recognise him and he wouldn't recognise me. I don't know to this day who he is, I don't know his name. It was quite a nice flat, not amazing, but he must have been quite wealthy, and from his body I think he was youngish, probably mid-thirties, and in quite good shape. I wouldn't do this today. It was a stupid thing to do, and I don't know why I did it then. I was going through a stage where I was very sexually adventurous.

He rang me the next day and said that it had been amazing. I'd lived out his sexual fantasy so he would provide mine, whatever it was. I'd told him the one about the two Japanese ladies giving me a massage when we'd talked originally about our fantasies, and he now said that he didn't know any Japanese ladies,

93

but he knew two Thai ladies who he could get to live out my fantasy. But I said no, I didn't want to do it, and I didn't want to see him.

I didn't want any more to do with it, because I was so disappointed. I had just assumed that I would get hooked into his fantasy and enjoy it, but I didn't. I wasn't repulsed by it, it just did nothing for me, so I didn't want to pursue it any further. It was a disappointment, but I'd learnt that while I like to fantasise, I don't want to live them out.

Alex aged 27

I was brought up speaking Greek as my first language, which I think is quite important in terms of sexuality and how I came to play around with different ideas of sexuality. I come from a very middle-class background and came out when I was seventeen, though actually I didn't have any sexual experiences until I was twenty-one. My sexual experiences started here, and I think that's important, because they've always been experienced in a language that is not my mother tongue, and my fantasies have incorporated that to a great extent.

My actual sexual relationships have always been with women, but that's not the case with my sexual fantasies. I think that while the fantasies have changed quite a bit in the last two years, one thing that has always shaped them is the language, which gives distance. The foreign language is a filter that allows me to be less censorious, so I can fantasise about a much wider spectrum in English than I would in Greek. Another very important thing for me is living in the city. I've been living in London for the last few years, and that again gives me anonymity, being part of a large lesbian scene where there is the possibility to change partners, whereas in smaller towns the possibilities are far more limited.

The fantasies I have now tend to turn very much around sado-masochism. I think I can trace these fantasies back to my childhood, when I was seven or eight, before they were even gender specific. Even now these fantasies are not particularly gender specific. The important thing in them is the sexual position, and the power games, as opposed to the anatomy. They almost always involve props and sexual games, and they are based around a scenario of anonymity. I never fantasise about people I fancy, or about a partner I'm with, or anything like that. It's just a body. The thrill of anonymity and being in a situation where I'm powerless is what turns me on. I'm manifestly powerless, at the bottom, which in S & M vocabulary means submissive, but in fact the power is with me at all times as I am in control of the fantasy, and because it's all programmed to give me pleasure.

Recently I've started having fantasies in a gay male scenario. I would say that I'm gay male identified, because I'm fascinated by the codes of seduction and sexual practice that are set up by

95

gay men, more than by the traditional image of lesbian seduction; also because in a gay male context, with practices like cottaging, sex in men's toilets, anonymity is important. Some of my fantasies take place in a gym (I work out), or a club (I like music), and I'm being eyed by someone I don't know across the floor. I have no verbal contact with them at all, just eye contact, and I'm being made to understand what this person wants from me, and overpowered by the person's desire, and set up to perform whatever they want me to perform. And I'm being asked to service them, to fuck them and things, and I have my clothes taken off, and I'm fucked, penetrated. But the important thing is not so much that I'm being fucked or penetrated, but the fucking is the manifestation of the power over me.

The fantasy could even take place in the toilet, where I could be forced to strip and then to service them, or to bend over and be fucked. And the idea is to push my limits beyond what I assume is my tolerance, and also to test my pain limits. I'm very interested in my pain limits, and when I'm having sex I'm very much into pain, particularly as it is inflicted on me and the kind of intensity that can bring, which is an intensity beyond fucking itself. It's a way of extending sex. Sometimes in the fantasy there's more than one woman, sometimes there are men, but when there are women it is important that the women are wearing leather, wearing strap-ons, and presumably carrying whips, clamps and other implements. One thing that turns me on is the absolute sense of being overpowered, but also the sense that what is overpowering me is not just a person but is also an instrument. It's not just a body that makes contact, but there is a body, another body and something in between which is a foreign body, an instrument made of rubber or leather. I'm being hit, held down and fucked, and the fact that the dildo is an object rather than a hand or a dick is a great turn-on for me.

As far as women are concerned, that's the sort of fantasy I have. I'm very rarely on the top in these situations. There are other fantasies where I fantasise about being a voyeur, but usually what I'm looking at is a scenario involving gay men. Again it's a scenario involving extreme pain. Even in my fantasies I'd be very reluctant to witness a scenario involving women in extreme pain, but when men are concerned, censorship does

96

not arise. Another fantasy involves being a voyeur in a situation where a man is topping another man and whipping them to the point of severe pain, and perhaps cutting them, fucking them, fisting them and so on. I'm just watching these scenes, but sometimes I can participate as well – but at the 'top' in that situation.

Other fantasies I've started having recently involve men, but again specifically a gay male scenario. although the women don't have to be of a particular body type (though I like them to be muscular), with men they have to be extremely over the top, beautifully built like bodybuilders and usually white, and in their twenties. I often fantasise about being able to take over a gay man who's strapped down on a bench or a table and unable to move, so I can play with him as if he's a complete object. He has no say at all in what happens to him. And his pleasure, which occurs, is something that I'm stealing from him. So basically there's a dick to play with, it's attached to a body, but that body is completely immobilised, and it has to be absolutely beautiful.

When I'm actually having sex I do practise penetration both ways, on me and the person I'm with, but in the fantasy it's always excessive. It's always more than is anatomically possible to take, and everywhere as well: anal fucking, fisting, vaginal fucking, oral, everything that you could possible imagine and all at once if possible, with a number of different people. I'm being held down by a group of women who proceed to penetrate me. The whole emphasis is on them breaking the barriers, so that in the end I really like it, and I have to admit that I really like it, which is a kind of humiliation.

As far as safe sex is concerned, I know in fantasy it doesn't matter whether there are barriers, but nevertheless I think there is an element of censorship which has penetrated within my fantasies as well. Although I know in my head that it doesn't matter if there is a barrier or not, even at that stage I will find myself reluctant to have immediate body contact, particularly with men, without a condom, unless I've justified it to myself that I'm not coming into contact with the sperm really, so there's no risk of HIV. But there is also an attraction in coming into contact with the sperm at the same time.

Safe sex and the health risk is something that worries me in reality. And I think that with all the safe sex education there is an immense attempt to get all the fantasies, and the actual practices, to orientate themselves around liking and getting turned on by the barriers: rubber gloves, different shaped condoms, and ribbed ones can be part of the fantasy. This is now becoming very much part of my fantasy, and it's one more foreign object, which is something that I like. Toilets are a place for an ideal scenario, or an empty gym, especially to do with sweating out and being very toned up and turned on because of the effort it takes.

My actual sex life does turn around S & M, but I've never had sex at the same level as my fantasy, though it's something that I've always wanted to do. I have tried group sex once or twice, but I haven't really liked it. As far as women are concerned, I would very much like a lot of my fantasies to cross over with real life, and although I can't be sure what would happen, I don't feel that my fantasy is nothing to do with what I practise. They're not the same, but it's not completely detached, and my fantasy life crosses with reality more and more. There was a time when I would never have admitted that. But now things like S & M top/ bottom situations and fetishism are more and more part of what I want. I still haven't had sex with men in my life but it is something that I would very much like to do, but again there is the understanding that they would be gay men. The reason for this is that a gay man's desire is for other men, and to get their desire turned towards me is in a way like they're desiring me as if I were a gay man as well, and that is also what turns me on.

I like queer fantasies, queer as in gay and lesbian together. I think these fantasies are a good description of my sex and fantasy life over the last two years.

THE INDEPENDENT
CAREER WOMAN

The Independent Career Woman

Of the four women who discuss their sexual fantasies here, two are academics and two work in business. They are all busy, independent women for whom sex and sexual imagination are an important part of their lives.

Penny, an extremely beautiful half-caste girl, is a fashion buyer at a large department store. She feels she is sexually inexperienced as she has only had two partners, but is able to talk openly with her lover about her fantasies in which she participates in bisexual love-making.

Deborah, a lecturer at a northern University, also came from a sexually repressive background. She enjoys her sexuality, and takes a very analytical and positive attitude to its development. Defining herself politically as a lesbian, she also has sexual relations with men and fantasises about both men and women.

Tall, elegant Katherine, in her sleek city suit, works for a firm of Management Consultants, but conversely she feels that her positive approach to her sexuality was inspired by the fact that she grew up in the countryside, a farmer's daughter. She is single but has a steady boyfriend and follows his lead in sexual fantasy. Together they talk through sexual fantasies as they make love; this for her is a major part of his appeal.

Mary, a teacher, fantasises mainly about women, and now has women lovers. At thirty-one, she has a ten-year-old child and brings her up alone.

Penny aged 30

My family were quite open about sex. Everybody was always wandering around in the nude. And questions were always answered honestly.

One thing that did have a significant affect on me was that I found my father's porno magazines, and I used to read through them from the age of seven. I used to discuss these with my friends, female friends, and we began to experiment with things like touching each other in different places to see how it felt. We often made each other come. At a friend's house we found much more hard core magazines that her father kept hidden, they contained pictures of things like couples actually having sex, and bondage. My father's magazines were just things like *Penthouse* in which I saw what I thought were quite glamorous depictions of women. I loved the pictures of these glamorous and naked women and used to imagine myself as one of them. I had orgasms quite young, I think about fourteen, when fantasising about these women.

When I was sixteen or seventeen I suddenly felt bad about my fantasies being dependent on pornography. I became politically more aware and began to look elsewhere for expressions of women's sexuality. So I started to read Anais Nin, her fantasies appealed to me in that they were quite fairy-tale like, there was a lot in them about what people were wearing, a lot of glamour, and also abdicating responsibility and being taken. Beauty rather than the ugliness and seediness of the pornographic magazines.

I've only ever been out with two men, one for ten years and more recently the other for three years. Sometimes I feel I've missed out a bit sexually because of the monogamy. In my first relationship I felt very safe and secure because it lasted so long and we knew each other so well. We were able to talk about our fantasies while we were having sex. I always fantasise about things I wouldn't actually ever want to do, but I find it exciting to take risks in my imagination. Usually I have bisexual fantasies, with more than one other person involved.

My fantasy takes place in a harem. I am lying down on some cushions in a big empty palace room, two girls come in beautifully dressed in corsets intricately spun with golden thread. They begin to touch and stroke my naked body, touching my bum and stroking softly between my legs, then one starts to kiss me between my legs. This goes on for some time, slowly building up, one sucking my nipples, one between my legs. I am aware that I am being prepared for the man who's going to take me later.

A man comes in, I don't know who he is, he comes in and I have to go down on him, the girls are still there licking and sucking. He dismisses them. And then we have full sex. Later he calls in another man to join us and then the two girls come back and we have an orgy. I'm always the central focus of the fantasy, everyone is always doing things to me. A lot of my fantasies end up with two men as well.

Another of my regular fantasies is one where I'm making love with a girl – which is something that I've never done – and a man is watching us. He gets really excited and wants to get involved. My fantasies are very detailed and in a way quite real to me, they always make me come. I use them specifically if I'm masturbating.

Deborah aged 31

Sexual fantasies have been an important part of my sexual growth, because in some ways I developed quite late sexually. I grew up in quite a repressive and prohibitive environment. One of my earliest memories is of sitting on the floor looking at myself, and my brother running next door and getting my mother to come in and say, 'Don't touch yourself, don't do that, that's disgusting!' It was very much the sort of environment where sexuality wasn't expressed or acknowledged.

I started sexual relations when I was seventeen, which is not that late. I obviously experienced sexual desire then, because I got into those relationships, but I tended to focus my attention on my partner and satisfying them, and not on myself. I had amazingly little understanding of my body, its arousal, its responses, and so on. And I was sometimes left feeling quite angry and frustrated after sex because I didn't have orgasms. I didn't really understand why, or really know what an orgasm was. I didn't know what I was missing. The men that I was sleeping with also either didn't notice or didn't know what to do.

When I say late sexual development, I mean that it took me a long time to start to understand my own body. I think I was twenty-one before I saw my clitoris for the first time, actually looked and found it and was aware of it as something. It makes me very angry when I think about the conspiracy of silence around the clitoris, and women's sexual pleasure. When you do sex education at school, you do biology and you're shown diagrams of the vagina, but the clitoris is not marked out because it's not to do with reproduction, it's just there purely for your pleasure. It's not mentioned, and I don't think I had very much sense of what it was and what it could do, the remarkable potential of it.

I had my first orgasm when I was twenty-six. I'd been getting to the point where I thought I was just frigid, and I thought maybe it doesn't matter that I don't have orgasms. But finally I made a concerted effort with the aid of a vibrator and some pornography and these very explicit feminist guides to orgasm, which I found very encouraging and supportive. The things that I'd been reading in ordinary women's magazines were far too

104

vague to be of help. What I really needed was something very explicit that really encouraged me to think, yes, I can do it. I remember thinking that it was just totally wonderful, it was really amazing and wonderful to have orgasms. And now I would never believe people who say that it's not important for women to have orgasms.

There's often that line taken in women's magazines when women write in and say they don't have orgasms, and they're told, well, you can get lots of other things out of sex, which is true in a sense – you don't have to have an orgasm every time – but if you never have an orgasm you're really missing out. I can't think of a sensation that I enjoy more than orgasm. I masturbate quite a lot, four or five times a week, and it's still – after four or five years – an exciting thing to do. I get a lot of joy out of the possibilities of my body.

To get into a sexy mood I think about women. I came out at twenty-five and fell in love with a woman and had a relationship. And I still view that as a fantastically liberating experience, to have a relationship with a woman. The first time I kissed a woman I realised what a kiss could be, the erotic possibilities of it, in a way that I didn't experience with men. I think that what lesbianism offers me sexually is a validation of my body. When I've had oral sex with men it's never been very good. In a way it's not just a question of technique, though in a way it is, because they don't know quite what to do and they don't have the same understanding, but it's also that they somehow communicate a discomfort about your body and about your cunt. They seem to communicate being unsettled by it, whereas with a woman what I get of course is a truly positive and validating attitude to my body. I feel loved and accepted in a quite a special way, and I'm able to offer that in return. Gay relationships make a lot of sense to me – women sleeping with women and men sleeping with men – because who understands how your body works better than someone who's got the same body as you?

Men in reality never used to live up to the fantasies I had about them, whereas in some ways having sex with women was as good as or better than the fantasies I had about them, which was quite exciting for me.

I think fantasy is something that has developed over the

years. I did have quite long periods when I was celibate and doing quite a lot of thinking about my sexuality and trying to understand it. I did a lot of reading, and thinking, and that's where books like Nancy Friday's came in, because they made me think that it was OK to have these fantasies and to allow myself to develop them and work on them, as opposed to just having a fleeting thought that you put aside because you feel a bit guilty about it. So for me it's an ongoing process that's still developing.

To get into a sexy mood I would be more likely to think about a woman than a man. I like just to imagine the way a woman's breasts feel or the wetness of her cunt. That would make me feel turned on sexually, and all the softness of a woman's body is very erotic. I still do have good casual sex with men, because I do find their bodies attractive in some ways, though I identify myself as a lesbian politically, because that is my culture and my community, and very much my social and political identity.

The irony is that there are a lot of lesbians who fantasise about having sex with men, or even on some occasions sleep with men, but that doesn't mean that they aren't lesbians and aren't committed to their lesbian identity. For me that label is as much about the ways in which society oppresses and excludes a whole group of people because of the choice of sexual partner that they make. For me, being a lesbian is a statement, but I'm clear there is a separation between that political identity and the things we fantasise about. I think that because we have heterosexuality thrust at us from such an early age it's quite easy to have short-term, not very deep relationships with men, whereas with women I have really deep, long-lasting, really romantic attachments. I haven't learnt to have casual sex with women yet.

My newest resolution with men is that if I carry on sleeping with them as a lesbian, and they're attracted to me partly because they know I'm a lesbian, then I'm going to respond partly by fucking them in a queer way. So I'm more likely to fuck them up the arse than I would have done in the past, because I think it's very important for me to experience being penetrated and to come to terms with their own homosexuality. Quite often I think men are denying that aspect of themselves, but acting out the fantasy in a way by sleeping with me as a lesbian. So I'm bringing it home a bit more closely to them.

I always need fantasies to come. To actually have an orgasm I usually have fantasies of a sado-masochistic variety. I've read Freudian analyses of fantasies which see them very much as the expression of forbidden desire and the punishment for it, both in the same moment. You probably could read my fantasies in that way, reaching back into my childhood and that parental repression; also just the social situation of a woman in society trying to express herself when there still isn't a lot of space given to women's autonomous sexuality, so maybe it hints at that. My interest in my own fantasies – and part of my brain and mind is still engaged in the fantasies even while I'm having them – isn't so much that aspect of it, but it's the way identity can shift in the fantasy between bottom and top, being the punished and the punisher. In the fantasy you can switch between those roles incredibly easily, and that's a central part of the pleasure of it, this idea of sado-masochism being like a kind of theatre, a play of power in which the roles change, in which they actually become loosened from your other social roles, and you can experience a rapid shift from being powerless to being powerful.

In my fantasies I am both roles at the same time. The fantasies usually start with me being the one who's being punished, but at the moment when the punishment is actually being meted out I'm fantasising just as much about meting it out myself, which is quite a liberating aspect of those fantasies. I haven't yet acted them out, because they involve enormous trust and self-knowledge with both partners. It makes me very angry that sado-masochists are represented as being very irresponsible and violent. I think that's not true at all. There's a whole S-M culture which is extremely responsible and involves people who do have that kind of self-knowledge and insight and understanding and are prepared to entrust themselves and their bodies to their partner, which is a very beautiful and intimate thing to do. I haven't found that trust with anyone myself, but I hope to in the future, though probably with a woman rather than a man. I think I'd feel unhappy about doing that with a man, unless perhaps I was the dominator in the acting out, because there would be too much of an alignment between social roles and the play roles in the fantasy. Because men have more power socially, I would find it a bit uncomfortable to be in a sexual situation where they were also acting as the ones with more power; whereas with a woman you've got more flexibility around changing the roles, and gender and power are less aligned.

I have used fantasies to come with a male partner. Because I don't come during sex itself, the next step is for me to bring myself off after the sex has finished, and with a man I'd have him whispering fantasies in my ear that make me come, fantasies of a very gently S-M nature. I'm very happy for him to talk me through the fantasy, but I wouldn't necessarily want to try it out with him. Obviously the fantasies are pretty impossible to act out a lot of the time, because they'd involve athletics and things, but they are some sort of a guide to your desires and what you want. Sometimes it is a good idea to try and bring the two together a bit. If your fantasies are showing you that there's something you want very much that you're not getting in actuality, they can be some sort of a guide as to how you can bring some of those fantasy elements into your actual sex life.

I've got one fantasy, which is quite a long fantasy, which I've worked on for a while. I'm in a huge castle, in a very large room. I'm a prisoner, and I've obviously done something wrong, but unspecified, like try to escape or something. There's a woman who is a very important figure there, because she keeps checking that things are safe, so the safety is built into the fantasy, and there are about a dozen naked men, and she tells them that I have been sentenced to be whipped. She starts by showing them where it's safe to hit me so that they don't inflict any long-term damage. It's not a dank, dark dungeon, it's more like an office with a desk and carpets. First of all the men try out a range of different whips, just playing around and seeing what effect they would have. They're not hitting me hard. And then at the end of that the woman says that the bloke with the biggest erection will get to dole out the real punishment and fuck me afterwards. And then she pushes me over on the whipping block and pulls up my skirt. She's always there checking that things are OK. Initially I get whipped by these men and the aim is just to see me and make my arse go red and twitch and see what effect these different instruments have on me – whatever twelve instruments I can think of. The fantasy usually fades after about three, because I can't think up twelve different types of whipping instrument. My orgasm is starting to build at this point, so the point where I come is the point where the man with the biggest erection takes a cane or a whip and is hitting me hard with it, and it's at that point of pain that I usually am able to come.

Another thing is that the men are naked and so are also quite vulnerable. They're going to be inspected by this woman to see which of them has got the biggest erection, so in a sense they're in a slightly humiliated position as well, because there are going to be some who don't have big enough erections. So they are competing with each other.

My fantasy often changes at the point where the strokes actually get delivered – these are the points where suddenly I'm delivering them. So I've switched my identity from being the one stretched out on the whipping block to being the one who is holding the whip and delivering the strokes, so I don't experience the pain; what I experience is giving it out.

I had a dream some years ago. Obviously it had all sorts of meanings connected to the time and context in which I dreamt it, but it has stayed with me. It's developed into something of an erotic fantasy that I work over in my mind, as an expression of my sexual ambivalence. In the fantasy I'm standing at the bottom of a mine shaft, which is quite funny as well, because it is quite resonant both in the image and the words. I'm standing in front of a lift and I'm really excited, because down in the lift is going to come this woman, and she's going to be mine to do what I like with. She arrives, and she has very large breasts that are bound in clingfilm. I find this a real turn-on and I'm touching her breasts in great excitement, and as I explore even further I'm delighted to find that she also has an erect cock. She's got everything that I'd like, the breasts and the cock, but she is definitely a woman, not a man with breasts. The dream expresses the ambivalence of being a woman who loves women but also likes cocks.

One of the privileges now is that lesbians feel that they can admit to fantasies, which they felt a bit wary of doing in the seventies and eighties, and we can also act out these fantasies with dildoes. So in effect we can have everything, because we can have all the beauty of another woman's body and all the exciting aspects of that, but we can also play out the fantasies of sometimes sleeping with men by using dildoes and strap-ons and so on. I think that would probably be my ideal situation.

The best advice I ever got about sex was when I was having counselling in my early twenties. When I was a bit concerned about not having orgasms, the counsellor said to me, 'Sex gets better as you get older', and I think that's definitely true.

What it means to me now is that there are loads of things to look forward to, like at some point being able to come with my partner during as opposed to afterwards, and maybe more acting out of selected bits of my fantasies.

Katherine aged 37

I'm a farmer's daughter. I was brought up in the country, so we were more aware of a Lawrentian attitude to sex – that it's very natural and very beautiful. My mother was very, very strict, and anything like sex was completely prohibited, but not in a warped, twisted way. It just wouldn't be something you'd bring up; she was a little bit Victorian. Father was very free and liked women to be independent and strong and wanted us to be business women, not 'Laura Ashley wives'. I know that when I eventually went to school in the city I probably knew a lot more about what was going on than the other girls. Not that we were very permissive in the country, it was just a nice open attitude to sex. I hope I've been like that ever since. I've certainly had a lot of fun.

I'm single, never been married, never even lived with anybody, but I did have a very steady boyfriend for the last seven years. He wasn't ready to make a commitment – didn't want to make a commitment. I've just got a new boyfriend last year and I don't know how it's going to work out. We got off to a great start for six months, and now we're in a cooling off period. We both got scared and we both stood back. We haven't split up or anything, we're just thinking about it. He's great, great fun, and he's the one I want to tell you about. I don't have lots of partners, I like to have my one steady relationship. In between relationships I can go a little bit wild, but nothing much. I mean, four guys in one year's a lot. I've done a few naughty things, fun things. I think sex is fun, which I think we all do in the nineties. This chap I'm seeing is incredibly attractive. He's about six foot three and very beautiful, almost like Warren Beatty. His family were a theatrical family. His mother was very famous in acting, and he was in the film business, a film director. Now, we talk through our fantasies together, and my fantasy life revolves around him.

I can't really remember much about my earlier sexual fantasies. I remember having them at about five or six years old, and I can remember having them in my teens and my twenties, but I can't really remember having very strong or regular ones in the last ten years.

If I fantasise on my own it's usually about the last time I was with my partner, in fact it's always that. I had absolutely brilliant

111

sex with my last boyfriend, and we're still great friends. But this current man is very erotic, a huge ego, but he's almost godlike, very, very, very, very beautiful and he has very strong fantasies which take over my fantasy life. I couldn't believe it the first time I slept with him. He does everything Richard Gere style, as if you were watching a movie. Very few guys actually take the time in reality. He's very beautiful in his movements, very artistic, slow, very tender. It's great to watch it on TV, but you never actually meet a guy who makes love like that – but he does. The very first time we slept together he instantly started to speak his fantasy. Having spoken to other guys, I know that they usually do have a fantasy running. Partly because he's in the film business, partly because he's probably got to an age where sex just for sex's sake isn't terribly interesting any more, he actually speaks his fantasy out loud. He speaks it beautifully, as if he is compiling a movie, so I don't need to have a fantasy – he actually will create the fantasy for me.

He does it incredibly. He makes me join in – he'll prompt me, and he'll say, 'Do join in.' It's a lot easier than it sounds. He'll direct it – he likes to manipulate people, but in a nice sort of way – as if he's directing a movie. He'll speak his fantasy, and they're nice, they're good – usually threesomes, a third person watching us, or that I've gone for a massage, and I'm being massaged by a man, and he's watching me being massaged, and perhaps the man will start to make love to me. Usually my boyfriend will actually relate a story where he's gone to visit a girl and her boyfriend, and they've got very close, and the girl has started to undress him and the boy has watched. He likes to be a voyeur. He thinks that the sex on its own isn't enough for anybody; it's the fantasy around sex which is exciting. He creates the most incredible atmosphere, almost a euphoria, an aura, as if you were watching in 3-D. He just creates a Steven Spielberg fantasy around any situation, like watching a film. It's always nicely done, sometimes a little bit rough and exciting, and he can be annoyed if you don't join in. He's unconventional, not kinky in a bad way – things like three people, two girls, slightly dirty words, but not too out of the way. If you go to the movies you're not just going to watch light and colour and people moving about, it's the fantasy which surrounds all that which creates the enjoyment.

I fantasise, when he's not there, about his fantasies. He creates them so vividly, and they're much better than anything I could ever think up, so I can use his fantasies to start again. He'll probably use the same fantasies four, five or six times. My second boyfriend used to talk in fantasies as well, but he never created the life around it, it was always monotonous and dull and boring.

My man now creates a fantasy inch by inch, detail by detail. One of the best ones is that I'll go for a massage, and the thought of being massaged by guys is quite nice, and it's relaxing, it's lovely. The guy will rub my shoulders, and rub my back, and rub down to my feet, and it's a little bit hot so he'll take his sweatshirt off, and then he'll take his trousers off, and my lover will come into the room at that stage and he'll watch. He'll describe in intimate detail how the guy feels, and how he gets closer, and how he gets hard, and how he starts to touch me, very very close to the top of my legs, and how he starts to make love, and my lover will actually be watching this happen. I think he does these fantasies for me, and not just for himself. This chap is such a good lover that he does it from a woman's point of view, he does it to create maximum enjoyment for the woman. At first it was a little bit daunting, because he always tries to manipulate. It makes it more exciting that he is in the film business – they are very theatrical people, who can't always differentiate between reality and fantasy. He would carry out the fantasies in reality, easily.

I did once live out a fantasy. I had my first threesome last year, two girls and a guy. It was great fun. He would try to set it up again, do the reality every six months and then use that to create the fantasy, but I'm not so sure. He gets really angry if I don't want to do it, but he's the one who says that the reality isn't as good as the fantasy. I see the fantasy life as something completely different and he can't accept that. He cannot differentiate between normal matter-of-fact things and fantasy, he's tripped somewhere along the line. He's highly creative, like a poet or a writer, and there's just a blur when it comes to reality. Whereas with me, the reality is actually very good, and the fantasy is well directed, it's great, but it stung me a little bit going to the reality. I wasn't as cool as I expected I'd be.

I'm dead lazy now. I don't need to create my own fantasies, and it's quite good to meet a man who will create a fantasy for a woman. Although some women do it themselves, don't they?

Though I can't remember them very clearly, my early fantasies were always about two boys together with me. I've also fantasised about being a guy, being a man making love to a woman. I think that's a power thing, and it fascinates me to know how it feels. I'd just like to know for a day what it's like to make love to a woman. I'd like to have a chance to be in control. At the moment my boyfriend stage directs everything.

I do love being dominated. My previous lover couldn't do this. His former wife had been a 'Laura Ashley woman' who'd only ever made love under the bedclothes, and it took years for us to catch up to the level of my new boyfriend, so I did have to take control to some extent. It's quite nice to be able to be submissive now. I think this is something else that has happened in the nineties. Women don't really need to wear their power suits and shoulder pads now. It's nice to go back to being fluffy and silly and feminine, which I find I do a lot. And I find I do that in bed. Recently I've liked to be a bit more daring in my fantasies, but essentially I'm quite passive and feminine, not dominant in real life.

When I actually did the threesome 'fantasy', it wasn't as I'd expected. It was great to fantasise about it afterwards, but actually being with another girl and her boyfriend . . . It was fun, a giggle, we'd had a lot to drink, and we did it in a really good fun way, mainly with hysterical laughter, but it was really a let-down. I suppose it might get better if you did it over and over again. The first time you make love with someone new tends to be a bit of a let-down, but then it gets better and better and you want more and more, so maybe if you did a threesome once a week or every night you would end up really enjoying it. It took me till the age of thirty-five just to go over the edge a bit. But now with my guy in the film business he makes the most wonderful fantasies, and he brings them right inside your body. He's very unusual. The fantasies become my fantasies and I rerun them exactly as he created them.

There's one fantasy where he'll arrive late, and he's late because he stopped by to see a friend. The friend had a flatmate, and she's nineteen and she's a ballerina . . . It's always the other couple who draw him into it. He describes what she is wearing: leg warmers, leggings, something loose draped over her. They sit and chat and drink, and the ballerina will lie down just a little bit on the floor and her flatmate will move towards her, and my boy-friend will say that he can see that she's getting very turned on. The men are wearing just robes by this time and he'll say that he can see that the flatmate is getting very hard under his robe, and he'll describe that. And he can see that she's getting very wet and they'll start to caress each other, and she'll look up at him and she'll pull him down towards her. And he'll say that she's got very small, pert breasts, and then he says 'I slip my hand on to her breast. Would you like to watch that? Would you like to watch that?' He'll be prompting me. 'Does that feel good? Does that turn you on? Would you like to see this?' And his cock is very hard. And he says, 'Would you like to feel it?' and we get very, very passionate and we make love very, very slowly all the way through. And then he'll go right through in every single detail as to where he touches her, and feels her and all the time encourages me to join in.

It never really finishes, we never actually fantasise about afterwards. My sister says that her fantasy is that the man is still there half an hour afterwards!

When I relive these fantasies on my own I hear his voice. He's there in my head. I only ever fantasise about my current partner. Sometimes I fantasise about him on a terrace with two blonde girls. When I tell him about the fantasy he always wants me to be there to watch, and 'will I tell them what to do and will I show them how to do it?' His biggest fantasy is that I will show them what to do. I have to order them to make him happy. At first I was scared stiff, but in fact fantasy-wise he's created a whole new life for me. It's more interesting.

Mary aged 31

I actually started having sex when I was fourteen, but I think that the idea of fantasy came to me much later. Heterosexual sex was for me very much about having things done to me, rather than actually taking part in something that was happening. There was a real switch for me in this when I came out as a lesbian. I've been out as a lesbian now for about eight or nine years, so it's been quite a long time, and it's a sexuality that I'm very comfortable with and don't have any struggles over. Certainly in fantasy terms there was a definite change, because I don't think I fantasised at all when I was having heterosexual sex. Since I've been having lesbian sex I do fantasise, so I think my mind has become more engaged with it.

For me this is about caring more about women. I never thought of the heterosexual sex that I had as being particularly enjoyable, so once I found a way of making it a much more enjoyable activity then the head stuff kicked in a bit more with it. The heterosexual stuff was much less pleasant. It was just 'nothing'. I didn't get very much emotional connection with it. And for me fantasy tends to be connected. Although when I was going through a bisexual stage I did have a lot of fantasies about women, and I've never had any about men.

I was at university when I came out, and had a child at nursery school. I had shifted geographical areas, from London to a small town, and this made it a lot easier. I came out about a year later after I came here. Moving to University was a very, very big thing, and not a thing that many of the people I knew had done – it was almost a way of changing who I was. I had already thought a lot about my sexuality before I moved, and how I felt different from the other women I knew. I knew only two lesbians where I came from and they were with each other, so there were only two lesbians in my world. When I went down to Kent there were suddenly a lot more lesbians around, so it became much easier than it has been for other people, because of the very supportive environment.

I think the fact that I used to fantasise about women when I was supposedly heterosexual was one of the things that made me wonder if I was a lesbian. I know that a lot of women do fantasise

116

about women and that it doesn't necessarily mean that you are a lesbian, but the fact that it started to happen a lot made me think, wait a minute. It was a sort of clue for me.

My fantasies have changed and developed over the years. At that point I just used to fantasise about things like kissing women and didn't necessarily progress very much further. But after I started actually sleeping with women they progressed a lot further than just kissing, and I did actually start fantasising about fucking them, because once the experience was there it crept into the fantasy.

What tends to happen with me is that the fantasies go in phases. Often I have a particular phase that might last for a couple of months fantasy-wise and then it'll shift into something else. Sometimes I have fantasies about real people. They're usually people that I want to sleep with and can't, for whatever reason. But it's not that common for me to have these specific fantasies. Usually I just see a body, or even bits of bodies that I remember. I went through a phase about a year ago of having lots and lots of breast fantasies. And very often it was just breasts rather than people as such. I had that quite a lot more than actually fantasising about real people. Also there's a difference between the kind of fantasies I have when I'm masturbating and the kind I have when I'm just walking down the road and go into a daydream – some of them are more deliberate. And I certainly fantasise a lot more when I'm not actually sleeping with somebody, than when I'm in a relationship.

I am in a relationship now and have been for about three months, and I've noticed that I've almost stopped fantasising, partly because I'm using my sexual energy in the relationship, and also because I'm masturbating less and that is when I tend to fantasise most. Before this relationship I had a period of celibacy of about three years, broken by the occasional one-night stand, but I didn't have a relationship for a considerable amount of time, and by the end of that I was doing a lot of fantasising. My fantasy life got much bigger, and much stronger. In a relationship, what tends to happen for me is that in the early stages there are a lot of new things going on physically, all kinds of different sorts of making love, a lot of variety. Once I get used to somebody and go into various set patterns of making love, then that's

117

the point for me where fantasy starts. it isn't so much about boredom as about familiarity. Safety also comes into it, as when I feel confident with someone, I feel safe in terms of telling them my fantasies. I could never tell someone about my fantasies if I hadn't been sleeping with them very long, because I would feel much too insecure. Somehow I go through a fear of thinking, Oh it's silly! And slightly embarrassing.

The scenario I fantasise about which always recurs is a kind of biker fantasy, because I use to spend a lot of time hanging around with bikers and I'm very turned on by things like leather, certainly leather trousers. There's an erotic charge around those kinds of clothes for me, so I love the bikers. The fantasy is a group sex fantasy really, about me and lots of biker women. I'm on a bed having lots of hands touching me all over, almost disembodied hands, so I'm being made love to by lots of people at once.

Leather is quite a macho thing, but there is also a sort of biker/dyke sub-culture inside that. It crosses over with the S-M culture as well, certainly in terms of the clothing, the particular sort of look. The leather trousers and things are sometimes connected to this scene and sometimes totally not.

Usually my fantasies are domination fantasies, with me dominating. The biker fantasy is not quite like that, though even then I'm not completely passive – I'm often doing things to other people as well as having things done to me at the same time. I don't feel like I'm in a passive, submissive state. My domination fantasies are not like S-M ones involving pain. I like the idea of tying people up, but not spanking, just tying them up and fucking them with fingers and dildo, rather than inflicting pain. I do occasionally think of this fantasy in relation to real people that I'd like to fuck.

I'm not at all submissive in my real life either, so I don't flip my personality when I fantasise. I'm always the dominant one. I like to fantasise about things I would actually do rather than things I would never do. Certainly my fantasy about fucking a woman with a dildo was a way of trying it out before I actually did do it. It was something that I've wanted to do for quite a long time and have only recently started doing. The fantasy was a way of trying it on for size, a rehearsal. I like to use fantasy like that.

I've never fantasised about someone tying me up, because in reality I wouldn't like that. It doesn't turn me on, doesn't work erotically for me. In fantasy I'm even more dominant than in reality. The bit of me that holds back in reality doesn't in the fantasies. Sometimes I pick out bits of real sex I've had and use them again in fantasy – replay an evening, or an afternoon.

I tend not to use fantasy very much when I am making love to somebody. I mainly fantasise when I'm masturbating, except in one relationship that I had which was a kind of fantasy relationship, as we didn't do anything else together other than have sex. She would arrive late at night and we'd have sex, then she'd leave in the early hours of the morning.

In my current, more holistic, relationship, the only fantasy I do have with my lover is that when I'm fucking her with a dildo, I fantasise not so much that it is a penis, but that I can feel what she is feeling. The frustrating thing with using dildoes is that you can't feel. My fantasy is that I'm fucking her with part of me, and I fantasise that I come, that it ejaculates, which often does make me come. I would like to be able to feel it, like I do if I'm using my fingers, so I fantasise about the dildo.

When I was first out as a lesbian I was very nervous about anything that would come near a penis fantasy because of that whole stereotype about lesbians wanting to be men, so I said no to the whole thing. Eventually I got much more comfortable with the idea of me as a lesbian, knowing that certainly for me it's not about wanting to be a man.

Five years ago I would never have dared to admit that I would be interested in fantasising about dildoes, let alone anything else, but as I've got more comfortable with my lesbian identity it's become easier to admit that that's part of it, because penetration is something I've always enjoyed.

The first sexual experience I ever had was with a woman, and I then blocked that experience for a long time. I've never gone for romance in any of my relationships. It's an erotic attraction I have for women which just isn't there with men. I've never been interested in men's bodies. My heterosexual experience was always more of a response to men wanting me than me wanting them, whereas with women the desire is on my part as well as on the other woman's part.

119

DOWNTOWN GIRL

Downtown Girl

Kym and Ruth both have particularly physical fantasies. Tall and skinny, Kym grew up on a council estate in a seaside town. She has very athletic fantasies which take place in the gym. She imagines she is making love to body builders, and that her own body is much admired.

Ruth, with her short muscular build and cropped hair comes from the rougher part of north-east London. Her fantasies are about aggressive physicality and punishment. She comes from quite a straight-laced family and yearns to be punished for the sexual guilt she feels. Her imagination veers towards the confused and violent. After our interview she tells me that she has many more extreme fantasies about being hit and in pain, but she will not tell me them. Her aggressive sexual fantasies are apparently rebellious – a normal rebellion against parental sexual repression. The two abortions she has had in her twenty-nine years have affected her badly and she obviously feels guilty and unhappy about them. One was quite recently. The first thing she said to me when she came round to discuss her sexual fantasies was 'how lucky you are' when she met my young son.

She was killed in a road accident a week after we met, when her car crashed through a motorway verge.

Kym aged 31

When I was growing up we talked about sex a lot at home. We sat down and talked about the birds and the bees, and we did things like walk around with our clothes off, and no one was very inhibited, though I never knew that my parents had sex. I never heard them or saw them, so I didn't think that they did it.

I don't remember having any sexual fantasies as a teenager. I think the fantasies only came when I got bored with sex. I got to the stage in my sex life where I began to want to deviate from the norm, to think about other things I could do; though you don't necessarily actually do them with the person you're with. And I'd been with the same man for years.

A few years ago my fantasies were all about people watching, men, just men watching and not women. Since I've been doing body building, Arnold Schwarzenegger has been featuring strongly in my fantasies. He is at the gym watching me work out, and he says things like, 'Wow, she's brilliant!' and then we get off together. All my fantasies are to do with bodies. They all look really brilliant, very muscular, handsome, tall. They are really beautiful and strong.

Now that I've got a baby, I haven't much time for fantasies, but generally it's gone back to being watched – lots of men watching as we make love. Usually I'm in bed in the fantasy and the men are looking through the window. They're a sort of sneaky, uninvited audience. But when I think they're watching I feel a bit guilty. I wouldn't really like to do my fantasy in reality. As soon as I think that the front door is open or the curtains undrawn I think, oh no, I must rush and shut the door, or curtains.

On the other hand, I wouldn't mind doing the Arnold Schwarzenegger fantasy, or acting out a fantasy involving wearing black stockings and stilettos. I have done dressing up fantasies, and I think they're fun, and make sex more interesting. I also fantasise about being tied up and being overcome. I never fantasise about being dominant over the man – the man is always dominant over me. I don't know whether this is because in the relationship I'm in the man is less dominant than I am; it could be, I don't know. But that's my fantasy, always being dominated by someone.

I can remember only bits of each fantasy, I don't really run through a whole story. I can remember fantasising about being tied up, and someone making love to me tied up, but it's never violent, just the general idea. I have thought about the idea of rape, but I couldn't go through with that fantasy in full. Though it is quite appealing, even in fantasy I couldn't bring myself to think the whole thing through.

My fantasies aren't always with my boyfriend. In fact there is rarely a face to any of the men, probably because I'm quite a selfish, vain person. I am the centre of all my fantasies. There is obviously someone there with me, participating, but I am the centre of attention. Even when Arnold comes into the gym I'm the most important attraction in there.

My fantasies are flashes of thought in my mind, stockings, high heels, rope. I dress up in black stockings and stilettos, and submit to the demands of a big muscular man.

I believe that you should be open about sex and your body, and in general people aren't. People are so terribly conservative, even my boyfriend – though he's not now, having been with me for years. At the end of the day we're all the same underneath, and my attitude to sex is a very straightforward one. I don't think you really need to have elaborate sexual scenarios in your head, when a good bit of ordinary sex can fulfil you. I think that it's people who come from more inhibited families, who don't actually do their sexy fantasies – because they're afraid to or for whatever reason – those are the people who create a bizarre fantasy life.

I was interested in experimentation more when I was younger. For instance, I fantasised about what it would be like to make love to a woman. But then I did try it – make love with a woman – and it wasn't what it was cracked up to be in my mind, so I'd never do that again. It was somehow really gungy, and like touching yourself. It can be an exciting idea in your mind, but once you actually go to bed with a woman you think, yuck, it's horrible. It's not the same at all. Though I think that half the idea of fantasies is that you should do them. After all, what's the point in getting off in dreaming about it? It's much better to actually do something.

My main fantasies are just about straightforward lovemaking

125

with well-built men. The focus is always me, my body, and them desiring, wanting me. I am very attractive and they worship me. I like to be admired, for people to look at my body and think, Wow! Perhaps as I get older and my body deteriorates I'll get worse, dismissing my mirror image for a fantasy. Perhaps I'm actually quite insecure, always demanding attention, with myself as centre.

So, I'm in the gym, lifting weights, wearing nothing but a black G-string. The beautiful, well-oiled, muscular man takes me. He's much bigger than me. The sex is very gymnastic, never in one place, all over the room, on the different pieces of equipment. It's very animalistic. I hang around his waist, moving about him as I'm very flexible, then we're up against the wall. He is ravenous and passionate and huge, so that I feel every thrust right through my body. And when I come it's with my whole body – we've both come at once and it's very climatic. That's how sex should be.

My boyfriend does have a very good body, and sex is brilliant, but I still fantasise and get turned on by the idea of other beautiful and desirable men desiring me. I've fantasised about lying in bed and having lots of men in the room wanting me, and coming to me, taking turns, one after the other making love to me. They're all watching at the same time and all wanting to make love to me. It is all amicable, a nice fantasy, but there is a tremendous feeling of yearning, yearning for me.

I've been in the same relationship for years and years, ever since I can remember, and maybe the fantasy is about the mystery of other men. That and the desire to be attractive.

Ruth aged 29

I talk to my boyfriend all the time about my fantasies. It's just basically because I'm trying to turn him on, and he's also trying to turn me on. It's also a case of bravado, to see how shocking each of us can be. I generally try and shock him, possibly because it's an insecurity and I'm trying to keep him interested by trying to appear very vampy or sexy. Also, I'm older than he is and more mature, his first major girlfriend. Though maybe I should say ex-girlfriend, but we are still sexually involved. I've had more partners than him, so perhaps I'm just trying to reinforce the idea that I'm more experienced, and even when it's a fantasy I often try and make it sound like it's something I've done with somebody else.

My fantasy is basically either what I'd like to do to him, or where I'd like to have sex. When I'm with him I always fantasise about him; if I'm on my own I could just be fantasising about various positions and ways to have sex. But mainly I tend to be thinking about him. He's Irish and lives in Dublin, so sometimes I do it when he's not there. If he's not there it might not necessarily be about him, because it might be a bit painful in that he's away from me.

I get a real kick out of the idea of having sex with him in a place where we can get caught, found out. There must be something voyeuristic in me. I fantasise about the idea of having sex in a train carriage or in the toilet or something, which could be exciting with all the jolting. We went down to Hampstead Heath once. I'm thinking about him a lot at the moment because I'm in love with the guy, so I tend to think about him more than somebody I don't know. I don't think about other blokes at the moment, although when the relationship wasn't very strong I did think about other men. So, we were on Hampstead Heath, and tried to have sex in the long grass, but some people came up and we had to stop doing anything. But now I just fantasise about forests or being somewhere out in the open air and we're bumping into a tree or rolling into a river. Or we could be in a train carriage in the fog. I keep thinking about the film, *Dance With a Stranger*, when they were having sex just by a wall, and I think about places where you can get caught, where part of the excitement during the sex is the idea either of it being forbidden, in a forbidden area, or else you're just about to be found out, so it's much more intense over a short period of time, which is really exciting.

When I'm on my own sometimes it's really hard to think of sex because I'm too broody and too pissed off and too frustrated that he's not there. So I do tend to block it out, but I'm really bored when I'm at work, so I do think about it then, it's a form of escapism. Again, it's usually the idea of having sex in a shower or a bath, or on the floor, very basic bog-standard kind of stuff. It could be the position that I think of, or the idea of being massaged whilst having sex, massaging a bloke and then having sex afterwards. It's all about stimulation, but nothing very unusual. If you're in a really good relationship it's something that you'd probably do anyway.

I come from quite a straight-laced family and that's probably why I have the fantasies about being discovered making love – the idea that sex is somehow dirty and forbidden. My family have quite a good sense of humour, but it's not a sort of sexy black humour. They're quite disapproving of my having sex, because I'm not married, and not engaged or in a nice regular relationship. I like the idea of being caught in the act, because I see myself as a sort of rebel from my straight-laced parents. Also, the idea of someone seeing me making love in a public place makes me feel attractive. It's the idea of them being turned on by it that's quite nice. I like to think of myself as really vampy, whereas in real life I have quite low self-esteem.

I am in fact quite an outspoken person, quite blunt. I don't know why I'm finding it really hard to think about sexual fantasies. I think about sex a hell of a lot. But I feel guilty and worried about it, because I've been pregnant twice and I've had to have two abortions, and I didn't want either of them. So in a way I feel guilty, because I think, Oh Christ, I could get pregnant again. I had one abortion this year and it's still very much in the front of my mind, so in a way I don't want to go the whole hog, although I do. And this is despite the fact that the other one seems so long ago that it is semi-blocked out of my mind. I don't know how far my sexual fantasies are intertwined with this, but there is a whole

128

mix-up in my mind about it. I like sex quite a lot. My ex-boy-friend spent a lot of time saying, 'Oh, you're only interested in me for the sex bit.' Which is very stupid, because I'm not.

I like vampy sex. I don't really bother to dress up, though he likes to talk about it. He'll say, 'It would be a nice idea if you were wearing stockings, high heels, and all the sexy underwear, and I could rip it off you.' He does like me wearing things like G-strings. I have got some of those, and I do wear them. We never seem to do the whole fantasy, but my idea of great sex would be to massage him with oil and then have sex and rub all sorts of crap into him like chocolate. But he's much too conservative because he's Irish, so a lot of my sexual fantasies occur because of that.

Sexual fantasies for me, when he's not there, tend to be straight sex, maybe sitting on a chair, or lying over a bath, and they tend to be very violent, physical. I like being taken from behind. I tend to fantasise a lot about being taken from behind – I'm not sure whether that's buggery or just being taken from behind. I like submissive sex, kind of self-punishing. When I have sex I do like it to be loving, but on the other hand I like it to be quite vicious, with lots of biting and scratching and oral sex as well, all as violent and as shoving as possible. I get aroused, but I find it quite hard to have an orgasm, so for me it has to be deeper, more intense, more violent, then I feel more.

I tend to think of sex as being aggressive and violent, though there is part of me that reviles that, because the guy obviously doesn't feel much for you if he's not going to be tender. What I want is much more intense, much shorter, so there is a kind of conflict as to whether I'm being submissive and being punished, or whether it's all right, just something that I enjoy.

I fantasise about the idea of coming into a room and having a raincoat on and nothing underneath it, and bending over and being fucked from behind, or lying on a bed and having sex. Or having sex with a stranger in the loo on a moving train without saying a word. Though I usually think of the one man, in a way the idea of casual sex is quite appealing. The idea of a train really does get me turned on, a very fast train going along rickety tracks. I see a bloke sitting opposite, a nod and a wink, then we go off to the toilet. We just have sex there, then he goes off in one direction, and I go off in the other. That is quite a recurring theme for me. The anonymity of it is appealing.

I sometimes fantasise about having lots of men in one evening, a queuing up system – though that sounds terrible. I kind of like the idea of having as many men as possible in the evening, and orgasms as well. It's all very intense, and the last bloke is my ex-boyfriend. I talk that one through quite a lot with him, because he fantasies about having two women fighting over him, one being me and one being another woman.

I still feel guilty about my abortions. The first time I was stupid, and the second time unfortunate in that I had a morning after pill and it failed. But the guilt in a way acts as a stopping mechanism to my sexual thoughts, because I think, I shouldn't be thinking about this because of what's happened. It's so stupid, you shouldn't have to have a regulation on the feelings or sexual fantasies that you have, but at the end of the day I just think, Oh God, I shouldn't be thinking about that. I should be trying to curb it in some way.

However, I think I've got past the stage of worrying about my sexual fantasies because I think people might not approve of me. My sexual fantasies include, to an extent, anonymity, or else they've got to be really intense and fierce and punishing. But then there is always that trigger mechanism that says, I shouldn't be thinking about this, it's bad, it's not right, or, I'll get pregnant.

HOUSEWIVES' CHOICE

Housewives' Choice

Maria, Julie and Jennifer all came from homes which were not particularly liberal sexually. In the homes that they have made for their husbands and children they have tried to be a great deal more open.

Maria, with her neatly pinned dark hair and skin tight leggings, is forty and married with two children. She likes to receive a lot of attention and pleasure in her fantasies. She feels that she has not been respected very much as a person in her life, and her fantasies are about lots of men finding her sexually attractive and being nice to her, helping her to enjoy life.

Julie, practical and pragmatic, also married with two children, has, on the other hand, only fantasised at quite a desperate time in her life when her children were young and she was tired. She believes it would be disloyal to her husband to go beyond this.

Jennifer is a generously-proportioned Surrey housewife who also teaches cookery. Her fantasies relate mainly to her relationship with her father. He disappeared completely from the family when her parents divorced, and as a child she never got over this. Her fantasies are never loving, always cold and calculating. 'I had a friend who swore that she always came when she felt she was so in love with her lover that she didn't know what to do with herself. They would tell each other about their love, and that made her come. That wouldn't do anything for me.'

Maria aged 40

My parents were extremely inhibited about sex and we never talked about it at all in the family. When I was of an age to have periods my mother put a pamphlet on my bed.

My dad was very shy, but he was also a bit confused. There was never any sexual abuse, but he liked us to do little personal things like combing his hair, and he liked being walked on, on his back. This made for rather awkward and difficult feelings on the part of my sister and myself. On the other hand he would rush from the bathroom to his bedroom with a towel round his middle, not wanting to show himself to us. There was no hint of abuse but there weren't strong enough boundaries there. Nowadays, with my children, I am very careful to keep things safe and within boundaries.

I remember playing games with my sister as we were growing up which were partially to do with learning about sex. They were mainly doctor and nurse type scenarios. I don't remember much other than that in the way of sexual fantasy. We were very inhibited.

For me there is quite a bit of guilt attached to the idea of fantasising, and a slight feeling of shame. I am very private indeed about the sexual fantasies I have; I wouldn't even discuss them with my husband. In fact my husband is horrified by the idea of sexual fantasy. He doesn't even like sexual images on television, he resents the intrusion.

All my fantasies tend to be very hedonistic. I like to imagine people doing things to me to give me pleasure. My most frequent fantasy is of a succession of different men doing things to me. They are sometimes strangers and sometimes ex-lovers. I like the idea of ex-lovers, as it makes me feel that I am surrounded by comforting people who have loved me and care. Occasionally in with all the men I imagine that there are other women there, not that I am particularly keen on women, but it is stimulating to imagine they are there.

I sometimes imagine myself being a type of prostitute who would be available to lots of men. I love the idea of being in a room and somebody coming in and making love to me, and then another comes in and makes love, then another. There are a succession of different men, sometimes a group. It's like a sort of gang-bang, but in a very unthreatening way. The fantasy is not violent at all, and I enjoy being the centre of attention.

I think the general themes in my fantasies are about me having the power, being in control. I'm able to have sexual relations with many men without threat. I've been attacked many times, and not respected all my life. For years I commuted on the train and was often touched up and humiliated. All my fantasies are about me enjoying myself.

Another fantasy that I have is that I imagine a really beautiful man on a desert island. He is willing to do anything I wish sexually and is terribly romantic and sensuous and sexy. There I am on this desert island and he just pops up from nowhere and swears undying love for me. The passion flows between us and I can't believe my luck. We make love seemingly endlessly.

Normally I have these fantasies during lovemaking. I'm too inhibited to have them in the cold light of day. I haven't told my husband, as he gets terribly upset by images. The other day, for example, we were watching 'Prime Suspect' on television and there was a scene showing the rape and brutalisation of a young girl, and this upset him a lot. Recently we went into town to the cinema and couldn't get in to see the film we'd intended to see. I suggested we might go and see a blue movie that I knew was on, as it's something I've always wanted to do. He was horrified, I think, and clearly threatened and upset by the idea that I did want to see these images of other couples making love and things. In a way I was a bit tongue in cheek about going, but he didn't discuss it, just said no, he didn't want to. He doesn't like the idea of having images to contend with.

Also, I get the impression that the idea of fantasies makes him worry about where it would lead. We both come from very inhibited backgrounds. And I think that there's also an element of me feeling fearful that if I admitted to my fantasies it would turn out that he would be thinking about something or someone else. If I knew that he was actively fantasising about some big, voluptuous blonde then I would feel less important. I have quite a low self-esteem and I need bolstering, rather than the knowledge of him fantasising about someone else.

I feel quite guilty about fantasising, quite disloyal to my husband. I'd be too inhibited just to fantasise freely, but it does come quite freely during lovemaking. It's quite sad that I'm too inhibited to verbalise my fantasies. Often when my husband and I are engaged in lovemaking I imagine great, powerful, beautiful horses mating. Sad not to be able to share that with him, but I couldn't.

Julie aged 43

My parents were a bit Victorian. I only remember seeing my father once in the nude and I was quite curious to find out what it was all about. The bathroom was a long room and my father was at the other end going to the toilet, and I can remember going up to the far end of the bath to see why he was standing up and I didn't do that. That was really just about noticing the difference in gender rather than specifically about sex.

When I was quite small there was a group of us little boys and little girls, and the story is that we did 'you show me what you've got and I'll show you what I've got.' It was under a blanket on a grassy verge and we were exploring our sexuality. Sex was never spoken about in our house. Even when I had my first serious boy-friend, a boy from the village who I'm now married to, I never received any advice. He was very good-looking, and I was about fifteen when I was sexually attracted to him. My fantasy was really only that I wanted him to touch me in different places. The idea and the reality felt good. But it worried me – should I have done this?

I didn't have full sex until I was eighteen, so my fantasies before that were limited as I didn't know what it was all about. I just liked the touching.

I've been married twenty years. When we first had the chil-dren our sexual desire started to drift apart, because you're involved in looking after young ones and your husband is work-ing extra time to try and keep the money coming in. So sexually you start to fall apart then. Whereas you used to enjoy sex once or twice a week, now you find that it may only be once a month. And I think that that was the time when I started to fantasise. I started to think of other people I might quite like to fancy because I wasn't sure whether the man I was with was really with me any more. Not whether he was having a fantasy, but whether he might be seeing someone else. It could be John Travolta, or it could be a friend's husband that I liked, that I would picture in my mind. I'd see his face. When my son was about a year old I did that. But I felt it was a deterioration in my relationship with my husband.

Speaking to my other friends, I found that the same thing was

137

happening to them too, and they were having similar fantasies. So I felt that perhaps this was after all quite a normal stage in a relationship. And the other being coming into the relationship in fantasy was certainly quashed by actual sexual activities. I just needed it to get going, because I felt that I wasn't stimulated in my mind, and it all became a chore. It must be something to do with your hormones at that stage in your life, or maybe tiredness. You seem to lose interest, but when I fantasised it brought it all back. I'd just think of someone who I knew and I'd get a craving, or a hunky film star who I could imagine I was with having seen him at the cinema. That was the only time I went through when I needed to fantasise. I was turned on by them at a time when I was beginning to think that I was getting frigid, and they in my mind wanted and needed me. All my involvement at that time and my energies were focused on my children, but that does pass.

Now I'm sexually very happy, and I know what stimulates him and he knows what stimulates me. We've been together since we were about fifteen and I married when I was twenty-two. Apart from a big split-up when I was sixteen for six or eight months, that has been it for me. There has been only one man in my life, and that is my husband.

For me fantasy is just a notion you put in your mind to stimulate you at a difficult time. I wouldn't want my husband to know, as he might think I wasn't enjoying being with him, which wasn't true. It was a secret, except from some of my girlfriends who were all at the same stage with children, so we discussed it. But we wouldn't say exactly what the fantasies were. We had all got to the stage where the thought of having sex with a man actually turned us off and we were beginning to wonder whether we were changing the other way. But we thought we couldn't be – we didn't want to be with women, it was just something that went through our minds at that time. It was to do with being busy, rushing about, not having time to relax, not having time to enjoy our lives.

I never fantasised while I was doing the washing or anything, only with my husband in bed. Rather disloyal, but I just wasn't stimulated. I couldn't react, and the only way to respond was to implant this fantasy person, who changed. It helped me then, but I don't need it at this point in time.

Jennifer aged 34

My fantasy has always been about my father. When my father left us I was about eleven, although he hadn't been around since I was about eight or nine. I can't remember when the fantasy began, probably in my late teens. It is really my main fantasy, or certainly the one that most springs to mind, as it is certainly the most bizarre. It's not the usual type of fantasy that people have about doctors and nurses, and headmasters, and that sort of thing.

I suppose it springs to mind as well because I always talk about it with my husband, and he doesn't like it at all, because he thinks it's unclean to think such thoughts, and I suppose that's why it's stuck, because its a dirty fantasy. Dirty fantasies definitely turn me on more than romantic fantasies anyway.

The fantasy basically is that it's my father who's molesting me and touching me, and that's it really, nothing more than that. But it's always my father. And he's the one getting all the pleasure out of it. I'm not getting any pleasure at all. I'm being made to do it. I'm childlike in the fantasy. I'm not in control, he's in control, though I think I'm grown up in the fantasy. I'm not quite sure, I think I am. There are a couple of images that are connected with it. One of them is that we used to be paid pocket money for doing little chores – if we did the washing up, then we might get five pence or whatever, and it's almost like this is one of the little chores I had to do for my father when my mother wasn't there. Sort of like, do the washing up: 5p, you sit on my lap: 5p, and it was just like a little job I had to do.

It's also connected with two other things. When I was very tiny – I must have been only perhaps two or three – an image stuck with me that I never forgot, and I don't know why it stuck. My brother had a swollen penis, and he came rushing into the kitchen and my mother said to my father, 'Have a look at his willy, there's something wrong with it.' And my father, picking up my brother, who was very small in his arms at the time, was touching his willy because it was all swollen and red. Somehow that image stuck with me. It was almost as if he was enjoying touching it, and that image has stayed with me. And I see that

139

image again, differently, of my father enjoying touching me in the same way.

I still think about this fantasy now, years later, and yet when I see my father and think about it at all I feel quite disgusted by my thoughts. It is just a very real fantasy. It's not that I would like it to happen at all, and when I see him I can't bear to think about the fantasy because it's just too horrible. But when he's not here it's very easy for me to think of it.

There was another incident that I connect with it as well, when I was between five and nine, something like that. I use to lie in bed with my father quite a lot in the mornings. It was a little ritual that our family had, that we used to get into our parents' bed in the morning and have a drink. My parents would have tea and I'd have a drink of hot milk. Quite often my mother used to get out of bed first and get dressed, and I'd be left in bed with my father, and he used to play a tickling game with me, which is something I still like to do. I still like to be stroked and tickled all over. And he just used to stroke me all over, and I used to like it because it was nice. I remember one day it seemed to me that he was going a little bit too far down below. He didn't actually touch me but I felt him tickling my knicker line. And I was very young, but even then I remember thinking, if he goes much further I'll have to say no, which is kind of odd, because I don't think I was quite old enough to be aware that he shouldn't. But for some reason that image stayed with me as well. It seems quite exciting now.

I don't really have an explanation. It's just these little images I have of him nearly touching me, and touching my brother. I'm sure it has something to do with the fact that my parents were divorced and he went away, but I can't quite connect that up. I didn't see my father at all between the ages of eleven and twenty-two, which is when I met up with him again. From about the age of eight he was rarely at home at all, so I only remember him as a very tiny little girl. But I was always Daddy's girl. I always wanted to be with Dad rather than Mum, and we were very close.

We used to spend quite a lot of time together in the evenings. I'm not quite sure why, or where Mum was, but I remember sitting on the sofa with my dad quite a lot, sitting on his lap being cosy. He always used to tickle me, and that seemed a very natural thing to do, but it was only later that it turned into something sexual in my mind.

I still carry lots of scars from the break-up of my parents' marriage, but they are perfectly normal in the break-up of a marriage and a family, and there are not any scars that I've never really been able to deal with. As far as the fantasy is concerned, it's always just been a fantasy to me. I was only really made aware of it when I told my husband, and he didn't think it was the sort of thing I should be thinking about. He suggested that it wasn't a healthy fantasy, and that I should really try and erase it.

Most of my fantasies are about forbidden things, but others are just normal ones, like being on a doctor's lap. You know, that the doctor decides he's going to examine you. It's quite standard, isn't it! I quite like the idea of lying down on a doctor's couch and he examines you and gets out all sorts of bits and pieces, tweezers and things. It's the idea of the cold metal that's quite appealing. It's nothing to do with romance at all; it's all in cold blood, somebody taking advantage of me. The fantasy is never to do with doing anything to the man; it's always somebody doing things to me, as if it's not my fault.

I quite like the idea of a whole group of student doctors. You've got a whole lot of doctors around the bed trying to diagnose what's wrong with you, and having a little prod at the same time, playing with you, that's quite nice.

I once saw a picture which made me think of a fantasy I've thought of before, which is the same sort of thing really. It was a picture of a snooker table with the light over the top, and the woman is lying on top of the snooker table with all these men around her and they've got snooker cues, balls, the lot. And this light is beaming down on to her private parts. It's the same thing again, it's men taking advantage that turns me on.

My fantasies are about being taken advantage of, but about enjoying it at the same time. I'm not letting on that I'm enjoying it, and also it's quite soft and gentle. It's not violent at all, I'm not struggling, I'm just passive. Oh well, if they've got to do it, they've got to do it type of thing. I'm just a slab of meat; secretly I'm enjoying it, but I don't let on.

I'm not very good at making up fantasies. I just have these one or two that I stick with. If I read a dirty magazine or a book it wouldn't particularly have an effect on me, though the fantasy about being on a snooker table was quite recent. I saw the picture in an Oxford art gallery. It was a rather daring painting, though I can't remember who the artist was. I think it was just the idea of the woman with her legs splayed apart on the snooker table so that everyone could see her, with the light shining on her, and lots of men all around. They were just holding the snooker cues, but you could imagine that they could poke her or do something.

I never fantasise about film stars, or some handsome man I may have seen, or anything like that. The sort of men that actually appeal to me are very safe, nice English gentlemen who wouldn't do that sort of thing anyway, so it isn't something I would want in reality. I suppose it's because my fantasy isn't to do with love or romance, it's just in cold blood, being used.

I'm sure they're not terribly healthy fantasies. It sometimes worries me that that is what turns me on, whereas I think that most women's fantasies must be about a man carrying them off, and reaching orgasm when he announces that he loves them, and that doesn't do anything for me at all. That's what always seems to be in the books. I had a friend who swore that she always came when she felt she was so in love with him that she didn't know what to do with herself. They would tell each other about their love and that made her come. I mean, that wouldn't do anything for me whatsoever, I'm afraid.

It's just cold meat that does it for me, something not very savoury. And I do think of my father when I'm making love sometimes, if I need to! If I'm thinking, I'm tired, I want to go to bed, just get on, I want a night's sleep – if I need to I use it. I always think anyway that I'm not the one who's getting the pleasure out of it, so even if I was thinking about my husband it wouldn't be me that was getting the pleasure out of it. That's what would turn m on; it would excite me to know that he was excited. I don't always think of this, but that's what turns me on more than anything else.

A big hunky man walking down the street would not turn me on if he didn't look honest or reliable, and yet in my fantasy life he might. But my fantasies are not about my being hurt or abused, not really unsafe. My father or a doctor are in fact safe images. The idea of bondage or rape frightens me to a certain degree, but my fantasy is not a frightening image.

I'm sure it's also got something to do with the fact that I wasn't brought up with any romantic or loving images, because I wasn't brought up in a loving family. My mother's a very un-loving person. She's never cuddled me or kissed me or said she loved me in her life. My father was very affectionate, but he wasn't there very often, and then he went. Everything was very cold in our family, so I wasn't used to any sort of emotional images or loving images. I used to think that that was the reason why I didn't have any loving images. It wasn't until I met my husband that I could allow myself to have soft feelings for somebody without getting hurt by them. When I met him it took me a long time to realise that I could have soft feelings without the danger of being hurt and that I could give in a loving way, but I suppose that's never come across into my fantasies.

I've never had any romantic fantasies. I always imagine most little girls having an image of Prince Charming coming along and sweeping them off their feet and everything being lovey-dovey and getting married. I was never like that. Everything was always black and white, straight down the line and quite cold, logical, never emotional.

Having a loving relationship hasn't changed the fact that my fantasies are still nothing to do with love at all.

THE OLDER WOMAN

The Older Woman

Margaret is in her fifties and Marion in her forties, both married with children. Margaret is also a grandmother. In general I think it is the younger women and not the older ones who are more able to express their sexual feelings easily. An increasingly open sexual climate and greater education in this area have meant that though women like these in their forties and fifties have greater sexual experience in terms of years, it is the girls in their early twenties who are able to talk openly.

Margaret, slim and girlish, fantasises about having sex with more than one person, and she imagines the scenario in different locations. She also clearly enjoys dressing up in pretty and provocative lingerie. She does this to excite her husband, but it is a fantasy for her too – she becomes confident and feels sexual when imagining herself in, or even actually wearing, sexy underwear.

Marion, who has worked long hours as a badly-paid nurse, is turned on by the luxury of the unobtainable. Popular music and film stars take her away on glamorous weekends to be pampered and spoilt. She fantasises about a life very different from her own. In the fantasies she is well looked after; at home she works hard.

Barbara, a striking red-haired divorcée, is more of a product of the Sixties in terms of her ability to express herself sexually. Via a manipulative relationship with her husband in what was an early marriage, she began to learn that she could take control.

Margaret aged 51

My childhood was never repressed, but I would never have seen Daddy without clothes. My mum probably told me everything that I knew, but when I went out into the world I realised that I knew nothing. It wasn't until I had boyfriends that I learnt all I do know.

I think I might have fantasised from when I was about eleven or twelve. Certainly I had some sexual thoughts, but as a teenager I think I was quite slow starting off, behind the other girls. Perhaps I had some romantic fantasies about the boys, that was all. I was slowly finding out about sex and what it was rather than having sexual fantasies.

When I was in my early twenties and my confidence grew, I fantasised about things like where you could make love, different people. I liked the idea of making love on the stairs, and I also thought it would be great fun in a ladies' dressing room in a shop.

Now I fantasise about being with a group of people. There are two men and women there. It would never be at home – I wouldn't like it to be at my home. It could be in a hotel or someone else's house. Most of the things I fantasise about are things that I could quite easily achieve. I never think of anything very way out, no extreme erotic ideas. In my group sex fantasy I could be at our other house, which doesn't seem like being at our home as it's more of a fun house. I think there would be four of us, two men and two women, or maybe just one other man with my husband, or maybe just a man on my own with my partner watching without the other man knowing, a secret. I've always imagined that I'd be in a very short skirt, and being quite a tease from there on.

I like to dress up in a feminine way. I think ladies are there to be feminine. We are there to have our pretty underclothes and our little skirts. I wouldn't ever fantasise about tying up and using some of the weird stuff you can buy, whips and things. I like the idea of dressing up to be pretty and feminine.

I dream that I might go off on a day out somewhere and I might meet somebody who'll take me out for a drink and a meal. Then we might have a wonderful evening, and it might go on from there, and then you'd have a lovely relationship and so on.

148

That's not specifically sexual, more romantic, but it does involve making love with a beautiful stranger.

When I was young, I grew up without many girlfriends that I could chat with. As I didn't have these friends, I think I used the fantasies instead of friends to explore, and in a way talk through, the early ideas of a relationship. I think I still use them in the same way now. Then as I've got older I've become more confident and more able to do and fantasise about more interesting things sexually. Mainly I like to think through the idea of dressing up. I enjoy wearing all my frillies anyway. It is a kind of a fantasy, as I'm aware that when I'm wearing these things I'm exciting my partner when we're making love. And I'm aware that I'm wearing the sexy underwear when we're out, even though I'm not actually flaunting it at that stage, I'm just very aware that I'm wearing it underneath.

Now that I'm older, and I still like to think that I could be found attractive, I think that fantasising is part of the whole process of dressing up and making yourself look nice in the hope and perhaps fantasy that you can still draw men's attention.

Marion aged 46

My parents never spoke about sex at all. It was a dirty word in our house, even down to the fact that my mum had a miscarriage and I didn't know that she had had one – my aunt told me.

I'm not like that with my boys now. We walk around the house with our birthday suits on. My mum and dad probably never saw themselves naked. My children can wander in and out of the room when I have a bath, nobody bothers, which I think is quite nice really.

In my fantasy life Cliff Richard is my Prince Charming, and Neil Diamond is my Prince more Charming – he is a little bit more muscular. I've always like them. Since I was a teenager I've fantasised about having my wicked weekends away with them. We'd go to some secluded cottage somewhere in the back of beyond, and there'd be romantic music, a nice dinner, people to wait on you. I'd spend the days in bed alternately with Neil Diamond and Cliff Richard. I fantasise about spending time with them, about doing the whole lot really, with them in bed. It's a real turn-on. I love Cliff's music anyway, so he could sing to me all day and all night and I wouldn't get fed up with him.

Mostly I fantasise when I'm on my own and have time to dream about a life of luxury with all these gorgeous stars. Will Carling comes to mind, because he's so lovely and masculine. I love to fantasise about being pampered by these lovely stars and imagining what it's like to be wined and dined by them, but sometimes I think I'd get bored – too much of a good thing. That's why marriages fail half the time, because people get bored. I could never imagine anything like that working as a permanent thing; I just enjoy having lovely daydreams about what it could be like. Some of these men are probably pigs to live with, anyway, though I should think someone like Will Carling would actually be quite hunky in bed – but I expect you'd love him and leave him after the fantasy wore off. I think my love of rugby has something to do with that particular fantasy as well.

I tend to fantasise about people who I can admire and like for what they do, so I like Cliff's music and fantasise about him, he's so sexy on stage. I think if I didn't actually like the people and what they did then I probably wouldn't fantasise about them. I

150

don't think I could meet someone in the street and start fantasising about them, because I wouldn't know enough about them. I like to know what they're up to and be able to respect what they do. I don't like any of the tennis players. I can't fantasise about them at all, they're too young. My fantasies are quite dreamy, not very explicit. Not every one is the same – they tend to be different for each person I fantasise about.

I fantasise sometimes about being able to dress up to be glamorous, to be able to go out and buy a hundred pound dress and not to have to save for it. I think that is because I've spent twenty odd years of my life in a nurse's uniform. I wear more of my own clothes now, and spend money on them, whatever the cost, because they can make me into a glamorous individual and I can enjoy the luxury. A nurse can be quite a fantasy figure for men. They tend to think that we're a bit of all right, but we're normal people, the same as everybody else. It can be very embarrassing when you get the male patients having their little wet dreams. It does happen and it is embarrassing. I don't like to be stereotyped. Men can be obviously fantasising about something while you're giving them a bed bath. Fortunately I'm at more of a stage where I can delegate now. I think men do fantasise a lot more than women.

Barbara aged 53

Within the family we were quite inhibited sexually. My father was a pretty sensuous man, very physical, but my mother was a Victorian of the first order. She'd say 'get away, don't kiss me, don't slobber over me.' They slept in separate, twin beds, and they were huge people, so I could never imagine them sleeping together – though it was an obvious fact that they had because they had two children.

I don't think I had any thoughts about sex until I was about six or so. My sister and I were riding bicycles, and my sister pointed to a condom in the street and said 'do you know what it is', and then told me. I couldn't believe it. When my mother was putting me to bed that night, and I'd been thinking about it all day, I said, 'If Adam and Eve were the first man and woman, how did they know how to fuck?' My mother screamed, and then shouted for my sister to come, 'What have you been telling this child!' I assumed my sister was in trouble. The subject wasn't mentioned again.

From that time onwards I was very aware of my sexuality, because my sister was very sexually and physically mature. At the age of nine she menstruated and she was tall and fully developed at eleven. I was aware of sexuality because my parents, particularly my mother, were petrified by her sexuality and what trouble she'd get into on the streets because she was also a rebel. So they sent her to boarding school, and I knew that it was around the issue of sexuality that she was being put in a safe place. I was aware of the fact that she kissed boys in the cinema.

When I was thirteen, my first vision of 'the act' was when I walked into my sister's bedroom one night and my parents were out, and there she was doing it. Fright, horror, anger, fear; I felt all sorts of emotions, and it looked most inelegant!

As a teenager I had fantasies together with girlfriends. We'd talk about romantic love. At that time I had been kissed and fondled by boys and started petting. We use to have girlfriends sleeping over, and we'd have fantasies where we'd play with each other as part of the fantasy, and there were no touch zones. One of us would play the boy and one the girl and there was a lot of fantasising about what you'd do and how it would feel. I had my first orgasm during this, just at the thought of the sex. Suddenly I found I couldn't move, because I was in orgasm.

When I was living with my husband, before we were divorced, I used to fantasise that I would be doing the drudgery and housework and then he would come home from work and come up behind me and start playing with me without announcing himself. Before I got married there was always a lot of foreplay which I found very exciting, the idea of whether it was going to happen or not. When I got married it was par-for-the-course that it would culminate in penetration and his orgasm, and it became very unexciting. In fact, though, it was probably a combination of going on the pill and the lack of excited uncertainty, and so from the beginning I didn't enjoy sex with him and would fantasise during sex about other men. There was always a lot of fantasising about foreplay because I found it so exciting, but the fantasy never got as far as penetration because I didn't find it very satisfying at that time. This was when I was a 'young married' in my early twenties – the first time I began to enjoy penetration was when I was about twenty seven or so.

I didn't have to fantasise very much in my marriage because my husband was kinky, and he did a lot of fantasising, both verbal fantasising and actually wanting to act it out. I, being the good wife, acted out a lot of stuff with other people. It was all in my head about how it was supposed to stimulate us into having a better time, this is what he had convinced me, but in actual fact he was just getting off on the other stuff. He'd say, 'this is good, it'll get us all worked up and then we'll come back to our own partners and we'll do "it"'. But in fact what would happen was that there was a point at which I could see that he wasn't coming back, so I used to walk out. What then happened, I don't know, but I used to get out of there. The culmination of other people wasn't what I was after. This was all about male manipulation.

Since I've been divorced I've fantasised a lot, and the fantasies have changed over the years. At first I'd have the sort of fantasies where I'd see someone and then fantasise about how it could be with them. But I would actually carry my fantasy through. After I'd finished having my fantasy I would actually go out and get that person. I was used to it from my husband, he used to talk me into fantasies and then present me with them. He

153

had told me that if you have a fantasy, or if you desire somebody, and you are a woman and you're not absolutely unattractive, if you put the proposition to a man, no man will refuse you. And in my experience no man does, all you have to do is present him with it and there you are, you've got it. So if I see a guy in a situation, for example when I was at a lecture and it went on and on, by three o'clock I was right bored so I started fantasising about the lecturer. At the end of the afternoon I went down to the front of the auditorium and gave him my name and phone number at work and said give me a call. So he gave me a call and that was it, we were off. It's not very fulfilling though, the fantasy is always better than the reality.

More recently – because I'm not as sexually active as I used to be, probably because of things like AIDS, my age and because I was in a four year monogomous relationship – I find that my fantasies are mostly about the sexual adventures I had in my earlier life. These are mainly to do with the really nice sexual encounters that I had, the particularly gorgeous men or the particularly unusual event, or anonymous incidents. They are unobtainable now because I'm not now who I used to be. I do still love the idea of one-off anonymous encounters, though, and if I'm away on my own for example then I suppose I still do these things, but generally I like to fantasise about actual events like these in my past. I don't know whether it's actually fantasising or reminiscing, but I suppose it is fantasising because I use them when I'm masturbating.

Recently I made a resolution, a mind-shift, that this is not a satisfying way to live. Now I'm trying to convince myself to believe in romantic love again. I think a lot of this has to do with the fact that I wasn't really able to share my life with anybody while my children were being brought up. I was very selfish about that, or perhaps I didn't have enough trust in anybody else to really let them in. Now that my children are going out into the world I think that I should open myself to the possibilities of a romantic involvement that goes beyond the short term. I'm really thinking I'd like to connect properly with a man, rather than playing with sex, or playing with company.

The fantasy that is at the forefront now is about getting back into the most successful physical and emotional relationship that

I've had, and having really romantic loving sex with that person rather than antics and gymnastics. Because this was such a good physical relationship, the thought and the memory of how it was – it just fitted properly together, the chemistry was right and the timing was right, and the emotional caring and the nice words that went with it – it surprises me that that is the fantasy now. I think that's because I've not allowed myself all that loving side of a relationship, so it has become the really fulfilling fantasy.

CONCLUSION

Conclusion

Life can be seen as a balancing act. In our sex lives, as in other areas of our lives, there is to some extent a subconscious need to even out extremes. The more successful and dominant we become in our outside lives, the more we need something softer and more nurturing, the opposite, to come home to in our private lives. Frequently this can cause conflict in our relationships, particularly when like marries like. A woman, for example, who appears very glamorous and outgoing to the outsider can often have a hollow place in her personal life.

The extent of sexual fantasy in our lives can also be seen as a product of our own physiological make-up, our hormones. It can provide a release from the stress and exhaustion we feel as people in the modern world. We also develop and explore many of our own sexual ideas through fantasy, using the fantasies both as a rebellion and perhaps even as a compensation for the person we really are.

Professor John Bancroft of Edinburgh University developed the theory that sexual fantasy is related to high testosterone levels, which influence sexual imagination as well as many other aspects of our sexuality. Effectively, the higher the levels of free-ranging testosterone that you have in your bloodstream, the more likely you are to have sexual fantasy, to have more sexual fantasies perhaps than other women. It increases the versatility in your sexual imagination, heightens the sex drive, and affects energy levels in general in other parts of your life as well.

Sex therapist and counsellor Anne Hooper considers this to be a very controversial theory, because it comes into conflict with feminist ideas about how we are sexual. 'One of the difficulties with even discussing sexual fantasy is the theory that we have

159

been trained by male domination in our lives to really only experience certain types of sexuality through fantasy, and that it's actually part of a male plot to teach women to fantasise.' She suggests that men's traditional need for female fidelity in day-to-day life fundamentally distorts the way women fantasise. 'What we should be doing,' she says, 'is to pay attention to women's normal sexuality and work on what goes on there.'

Currently there is also a strongly held political idea that really we should only use our sexual imaginations to fantasise about the person who is our lover. If you then go on to expand that to other people you are actually moving outside the real relationship, and losing touch with it. You are not just in a sense being unfaithful to your lover, but you are somehow being unfaithful to yourself, because you are straying beyond the confines of that relationship. And that is dangerous territory for its healthy survival.

Many women worry about their sexual imagination, often saying things like, 'Well, I'm very faithful, because I always fantasise about my lover or at any rate a blank face.' Within a relationship women will seldom admit to fantasising about another specific man or even a stranger.

On the other hand by being faithful to your lover in fantasy as well as in life you could actually be following a line that seems desirable and politically correct. There is a sense in which your sexual imagination is not your own, a notion that I find quite disturbing.

Psychologists confirm that the idea that testosterone is somehow responsible for a certain way of using your imagination is valid, though testosterone is in fact a male hormone, one which introduces and maintains male secondary sex characteristics. While there is no definitive work to prove the validity of this theory, there has been some positive clinical research. Gynaecological examinations suggest that women who have got what are described as immature genitals are women who also have sexual problems. Apparently they do not fantasise. Less testosterone could, it is suggested, be responsible for abnormal genitals, so the theory could well have some validity.

Use of sexual fantasy is also interesting because it points to the fact that as we have increasingly more powerful lives – and

160

women are today busier and more in control than ever before – we do still need an area where we can relax and be taken over and be mothered. And this is probably just as true of men as it is of women. 'The number of people you hear of who are actually judges or MPs who one also knows through various ways are into infantilism or being dominated by a prostitute, and in some ways become household slaves, is quite extraordinary,' confides Hooper. 'There has got to be some kind of common denominator, because they are opposites. Maybe men who are already trained at public school to become leaders need to have somewhere to go. Also it is incredibly stressful and straining to be a leader. One does need to let one's hair down, and that is the most intimate possible way of doing it.'

There were many women I talked to who had delightful fantasies about enjoying themselves, but there were also a lot of women who wanted what they called very 'dirty' sex – 'dirty' things like a man urinating on them, for example. One woman told me about how she was really turned on by the idea of the proverbial dirty old men in macs touching her; others wanted humiliation – to be taken over. Although these are not rape fantasies, they are in their terms 'dirty mucky' fantasies. The women were actually using this sort of language deliberately, as if they wanted to present themselves as the opposite of how women are traditionally supposed to be.

There are many degrees of fantasy which women have not usually admitted to; but they do clearly exist. We are brought up to be good, clean little girls, and it is therefore exciting to think that there could be a form of rebellion couched in fantasy that slips out within the context of the sex life. This is quite a progression on the part of women away from the old guilt-ridden fantasies of the stereotypical 'nice girl'. Though some women still fantasise on these outmoded themes, it is possible that perhaps some of these extreme 'dirty' fantasies are tipping the balance in a new, independent direction.

'It could be very much a rebellion,' confirmed Hooper, 'almost against something like potty training – "You mustn't touch that, dear, it's dirty." That potty training stuff can certainly move on to sexual touching. The number of memories that the women in my groups used to have about being told absolutely decidedly by parents at the ages of three and four, "Don't touch yourself down there, it's dirty," is practically a uniform experience; or it certainly used to be, and I would hope that it's changing now. I think that's a very interesting thought, that it could be their way of saying "I want to break out".'

So today, according to the evidence of my interviews, women for the most part no longer seem to be having the 'rape fantasy' where they are not in control. In general, they are not being submissive to men in the traditional way. These 'dirty' fantasies are about a sort of rebellious humiliation of which they are in control. Women are freeing themselves from traditional values and allowing their minds to wander with increasingly less inhibition on what was formerly thought to be forbidden territory.

Women's sexual fantasy can go further than this. In a television programme which explored the subject as part of Channel 4's 'Sex Talk' series, one of the participants explained how she often fantasised about being extremely cruel to young girls, little children, and that she did not like having these fantasies. It was brave of her to express herself so honestly, for they were very powerful fantasies about dominating children sexually in different ways.

These fantasies are of course the last thing anyone would expect of a woman. Perhaps some of us examine these possibilities in our imagination almost as a kind of safeguard. 'The great problem for those of us who have got faulty consciences is whether or not to act out the fantasies,' Anne Hooper explains. 'The Myra Hindleys of this world did act them out, and that is the great danger. The huge difficulty for women like this one, who have these fantasies, is in my experience that they become terrified that they are in some sense like Myra Hindley; assuming that they don't act them out, of course they aren't. And if they always know that they would never dream of acting them out in real life, it doesn't seem to me in the end that this is an issue, because this knowledge does show that you do indeed have a very developed social conscience. But maybe this is still a way of saying, "I'm pretty disturbed by the upbringing that I had; in some way it was too tough for me; I need to break out, I need to rebel."'

There is a wide variety of rebellious behaviour – the dramatic 'gothic' cult, for example. A 'gothic' is somebody who dresses up to look like a vampire, with a starkly painted dead-white complexion, and who appears in this style in their everyday life. 'Gothics' are very often members of the Dracula Society, and take their obsession very seriously indeed – often meeting in churchyards for late-night seances. It is of course just a style, and most young people will do it mainly for fun. But in common with the 'punk' cult there is more to it than that. They are also establishing their rebellion; most commonly, as with the punks, they are rebelling against parental values.

Another form of rebellion in fantasy reveals itself as the exposure fantasy. Making love outdoors was a theme that came up frequently in interviews, being seen masturbating, hoping to be caught. This again is about women being the blatant immodest opposite of what was traditionally expected of them. These women are excited by the idea of being seen to be sexy, of arousing a stranger.

Something that surprised me with the lesbian women that I interviewed was the sheer aggressiveness of their sexuality. Often when we think of homosexuality we think of men and penetration as the most aggressive side of this type of sexual activity. But I found that I was interviewing some women (admittedly without the wide-ranging intention of producing a statistical, scientific survey) who were describing their homosexual fantasies in unexpectedly aggressive language: 'and then I fucked her . . . '. This language, together with their descriptions of using penetrative objects such as dildoes, and involving practices like sado-masochism, I found very physical and provocative. What was particularly noticeable was that these images and practices appeared not only in their fantasies but also in their active sex lives. Although they were lesbians, they all referred often to penises and penetration with objects. They were, however, at pains to point out that it was not because they found a man sexually interesting, but that they enjoyed playing with them as if with a toy. They referred often to ideas that I would not have associated with these women before – restriction, restraint and humiliation.

The fact that they had 'come out', confronted and declared their sexual preferences, made them more daring and honest in the way they expressed themselves. They also had, so to speak, nothing to hide, nothing to lose, having made the declaration. They are less concerned with society's narrow prejudices. The non-lesbians found it much harder to express their sexual appetites. Perhaps too these women were able to give expression to their sexual aggression with other women because they trust women more. They would be far more passive and unadventurous if they were in bed with a man. Research done by Masters and Johnson on homosexuality showed the very different ways that men and women made love homosexually compared with the way that men and women made love heterosexually. The same sex couples were more able to experiment with each other, and felt safe in doing so. They also did not feel that they had to follow some kind of established sexual behaviour. The heterosexual couples were clearly following a pattern of lovemaking that they thought they ought to do. It could well be that if you are actually in what is not an established lifestyle – a lesbian relationship, for example – which assumes an established lovemaking pattern, you are able to experiment more freely. You can let go more and do things that are different.

'There are very many reasons for becoming actively homosexual,' Anne Hooper told me, 'and there are some people who are doing it who are really very angry with the heterosexual way of life. Maybe this is also being reflected in what one or two of these women talk about, not that there is anything wrong with that.'

She described a bisexual friend who made a video of herself and a woman friend making love. This was actually filmed as part of an education programme and what the two women did in their lovemaking was illuminating. It was rough and aggressive. This friend also held a sexuality workshop in conjunction with the film, in which she discussed why she had made the film and how she felt about it. She explained that people did not expect women to make love in that way, but that there was no reason to say they should not. For her this was a way of making love that had developed quite naturally and normally with her female lover. What she had found exhilarating was that her male partner had been able to accept her as a powerful woman as well. 'That was interesting,' says Hooper, 'in the sense that if you did that with a man, he couldn't possibly accept your inner sense of strength and

164

power. And some of that is to do with power; women can be much more powerful than they want men to know about, and they are frightened of showing it, probably quite correctly. Men may well be very, very scared.'

The other point about the lesbian fantasies which involve penises and in some cases making love to men, is that the women who told me about them are quite clearly convinced by and established in their lesbian lifestyle. I wondered whether this reference to a penis in their fantasy could be their method of showing rebellion – of being different, or even 'kinky', because their chosen lifestyle does not include making love to men.

One of the theories about sexual fantasy and sexual imagination is that it is a way of exploring things in safety, without actually doing it in real life. Perhaps heterosexual women who have fantasies about making love with women are exploring the possibilities, experimenting in the safety of their minds to see if they might enjoy the experience.

The idea of fantasy as exploring sexuality in safety links with the recent case of the MP Stephen Milligan, who was found dead at home on the kitchen table, naked but for a pair of ladies stockings and a plastic bag over his head. 'He was over-confident and overstepped the boundaries of safety. He also had to have extreme physical sensations in order to get a sexual pay-off,' pointed out Anne Hooper. 'The bag over the head does actually give you that extreme sensation. Some people think they are in control and are over-confident, and this idea would probably fit his character. Some people think they have a kind of magic life, and they push boundaries. It's something to do with confidence and also to do with perhaps not learning very sensible boundaries as a child.'

Many of the women I have talked to seem to fantasise about black men, often several at the same time. Katrina sitting in her giant champagne glass with several naked black men trying to climb in to make love to her is a case in point. Anglo-Saxon women with no experience of sexual encounters with men outside their own racial group appeared to fantasise about black men more than most. Ursula, aristocratic and in her forties, describes 'gorgeous dark foreigners' and her extreme fantasy involved them turning from men into wolves. Her imaginary men were not only dark but also foreign and fierce.

Katrina's view from the champagne glass is about being in control of all these exotic men. She is not really interested in being overpowered. It is a selective fantasy. She is selecting men from a target group of black men, which could well be her way of overcoming a deep-rooted fear of being overwhelmed. In reality she would probably be apprehensive about going to bed with black men, of whom she has no actual experience. Again this could well be a fantasy of contrasts, of opposites. In reality her boyfriend is thin and white; but her desire to be confident and powerful, perhaps the opposite of what she actually is, is expressed in her fantasy by controlling strong and powerful men.

Ursula's two fantasies, about exotic foreign men and men turning into wolves, also reflect the excitement and mystery of exploring opposites, and performing atypically.

Clearly there does exist a certain amount of traditional reticence on the part of English women to reveal and discuss their essentially private sexual fantasies. There is also a significant element of humour, passion and honesty.

I have included the age of the different women I interviewed, and to some extent have arranged their stories according to age, because I think that there has been a great change in the sexual climate of Britain over the last three decades. The younger women I spoke to tended to be more open and uninhibited in their descriptions than those in their forties and fifties, and even in some cases those in their thirties. Certainly many of my younger interviewees spoke much more freely than I as a thirty-one-year-old would have been prepared to do comfortably before I embarked on this book.

I was surprised and impressed with their candour. This may be partly explained by differences in education. The women in their early twenties would have been reading the uninhibited and thought-provoking articles of Anne Hooper and Irma Kurtz written when their mothers were pregnant with them. This remarkable change in women's expression of their sexual feelings today is a reflection on how these mothers have brought up their daughters to think about sex.